the hippocratic myth

WHY DOCTORS ARE UNDER PRESSURE TO
RATION CARE, PRACTICE POLITICS, AND
COMPROMISE THEIR PROMISE TO HEAL

M. GREGG BLOCHE, M.D.

palgrave
macmillan

THE HIPPOCRATIC MYTH
Copyright © M. Gregg Bloche, 2011.

First published in 2011 by PALGRAVE MACMILLAN® in the United States–
a division of St. Martin's Press LLC, 175 Fifth Avenue, New York, NY 10010.

Where this book is distributed in the UK, Europe and the rest of
the world, this is by Palgrave Macmillan, a division of Macmillan
Publishers Limited, registered in England, company number 785998,
of Houndmills, Basingstoke, Hampshire RG21 6XS.

Palgrave Macmillan is the global academic imprint of the above companies
and has companies and representatives throughout the world.

Palgrave® and Macmillan® are registered trademarks in the United
States, the United Kingdom, Europe and other countries.

ISBN 978-0-230-60373-8

Library of Congress Cataloging-in-Publication Data
Bloche, Maxwell Gregg, author.
    The hippocratic myth : why doctors are under pressure to ration care, practice
politics, and compromise their promise to heal / Gregg Bloche, M.D., J.D.
        p.   ;   cm.
    Includes index.
    ISBN 978–0–230–60373–8 (hardback)
    1. Medical care—United States.   2. Medical ethics.   3. Health care
rationing—United States.   4. Physicians—United States.   I. Title.
    [DNLM: 1. Hippocratic Oath—United States.   2. Health Care
Costs—United States.   3. Health Care Rationing—ethics—United
States.   4. Physician's Role—United States.   5. Physician-Patient Relations—
United States.   6. Quality of Health Care—ethics—United States.   W 50]
RA395.A3B5445   2011
362.1'042—dc22

                                                                2010044392

A catalogue record of the book is available from the British Library.

Design by Letra Libre, Inc.

First edition: March 2011

10   9   8   7   6   5   4   3   2   1

contents

To the Memory of
Ruth and Jere Bloche

acknowledgments

This book addresses a subject that has remained, for the most part, unspeakable in our civic life. Medicine serves many social purposes that are sharply at odds with doctors' Hippocratic commitment to patients—and with our expectations as citizens and consumers. Doctors control costs by forgoing beneficial care. They'll do so increasingly as health spending soars and cost pressures mount. Clinical judgment incorporates cultural and moral norms, including some that are bitterly contested. And doctors put their skills and know-how to use on behalf of national security and criminal and civil justice, at times doing great harm to individuals.

We ask doctors to do these things and then become angry when we discover that they've broken with Hippocratic expectations. Understandably, doctors don't like to talk about this. Neither do public officials, policy wonks, nor ethicists: Navigating contradiction among people's desires is a treacherous endeavor. To explore this realm, I tap the experience of those who've dwelt within it: doctors and patients who've found themselves caught between our incompatible expectations, as well as policy makers who've called on health professionals to compromise Hippocratic ideals. I'm deeply grateful to those who've shared their experiences with me for this book. Many have done so on condition of anonymity, out of concern for legal or other repercussions. I've kept the use of anonymous sources to a minimum, but, at times, I've found it essential to shine a light on issues and events that would otherwise remain unseen.

This book is a genre "hybrid"—a blend of narrative, investigative reporting, and scholarship. It's thus outside the box of what law professors usually write, and I thank my Deans at the Georgetown University Law Center (Alex Aleinikoff, Judy Areen, and Bill Treanor) for backing this project. My work on it would not have been possible without summer writing grants from Georgetown. I'm also grateful to the John Simon Guggenheim Foundation for awarding me a Fellowship for this project—and to Henry Aaron at the Brookings Institution and Dan Wikler at the Harvard Program on Ethics & Health for believing in this project and for hosting me during my Guggenheim semester. I'm indebted, as well, to Belle Sawhill in the

Division of Economic Studies at Brookings for additional support during my time as a non-resident senior fellow. And I thank the University of Chicago and UCLA law schools for their research support during my visiting appointments there.

During a lunch gathering at a tony law school a few years back, a group of professors argued over whether evocative writing, writing that told stories and stirred feelings, should be viewed neutrally or counted against candidates for tenure. Their shared premise seemed to be that readers' emotions cloud analytic rigor—or lack thereof. It's for others, not me, to decide whether the writing in this book evokes feeling (and does so fairly). But I'm grateful to two Georgetown colleagues, Robin West and Steve Goldberg (whose premature passing stole from our midst a sage and cherished counselor) for encouraging me in my belief that feeling is vital to knowing and communicating about matters that stir hope and fear. They encouraged me to take on this project and to stick to it. So did my good friend Elyn Saks—legal scholar, memoirist, and MacArthur Fellow whose courageous account of her struggle with schizophrenia did much to educate Americans about this illness.

For their comments and suggestions, I'm indebted to participants in workshops and conferences at the Brookings Institution, Georgetown University Law Center, Harvard's Law School and School of Public Health, Loyola University Law School, Stanford University Law School, Tsinghua University School of Public Policy & Management, the University of California at Davis Medical and Law Schools, University of Capetown Medical School, UCLA Law School, University of Chicago Law School, University of Illinois Law School, University of Minnesota Law School, University of Pittsburgh Law School, University of Toronto Law School, University of Virginia Medical School, and Wake Forest University Law School, at which I presented ideas and drafts that coalesced into this book. I'm especially grateful to Henry Aaron, Martha Blaxall, Allan Brandt, James Childress, Einer Elhauge, Richard Epstein, Ruth Faden, Judy Feder, Jacqueline Fox, Robin Hacke, Mark Hall, Dan Halperin, Peter Hammer, Claire Hill, David Hyman, Peter Jacobson, Emma Jordan, Allan Leshner, Jonathan Marks, Joan Meier, Thomas Naughton, Martha Nussbaum, David Orentlicher, Diane Orentlicher, Robert Pear, Lynne Randolph, David Richardson, William Sage, Sally Satel, Belle Sawhill, Carl Schneider, Michael Seidman, Alan Stone, Geoffrey Stone, Eric Stover, Sean Tunis, Greta Uehling, Ellen Waldman, Robin West, Dan Wikler, Susan Wolff, and Matthew Wynia for their guidance and feedback at various stages of this project.

I thank my research assistants, who played critical roles at all stages. At Georgetown, Anna Gorisch, Suji Jhaveri, Una Lee, Dan Lerman, and Devan Musser gathered and organized information on medicine's many social roles. At the University of Chicago, Shira Kelber and Rachel Beattie did similarly invaluable research. This project also benefited greatly from research support provided by Georgetown's O'Neill Institute for Health Law. I'm grateful to O'Neill Fellows Oscar Cabrera, Rebecca Haffajee, Katrina Pagonis, and Karen Sokol—and to O'Neill research assistants Toyin Akintola, Daniel Armstrong, Meredith Eckstut, Torrey Kauffman, Victoria Ochanda, Neil Rao, and Alia Udhiri.

Special thanks are due to Luba Ostashevsky, my editor at Palgrave Macmillan, for her enthusiasm about this book, her support when my confidence flagged, her deft touch with prose that dipped too deeply into the wonkish weeds, and her tolerance for my too-long delays. I'm also indebted to my agents, Todd Shuster and Eve Bridberg, for believing in this project. I thank Lydia McDaniel for secretarial support and Dianne Harrison Ferro Mesarch for her wizardry with Word, Acrobat, and a miscreant laptop. And there aren't words to convey my appreciation for the Georgetown law library's terrific reference staff, who tracked down hundreds of obscure sources, at times with minimal notice.

I'm singularly grateful to Amy Goldstein, an extraordinary journalist and an extraordinary friend, for her encouragement throughout, advice on investigative reporting, suggestions for cuts to fit space limits, and help in the final struggle against impertinent adverbs and subclauses. And I thank my dear friend Jacqueline Kraemer for her caring ear when deadlines loomed and trade-offs between getting it "right" and being close to on-time seemed impossible. For better or worse, I kept choosing the former. I'll be forever grateful to the leadership team at Palgrave Macmillan and St. Martins for enduring this choice.

Finally, I thank my last research assistant on this project, Anna Gorisch, for running the anchor leg—hunting down pesky citations, reviewing page proofs, troubleshooting the inevitable last-minute glitches, and otherwise superintending the ultimate stages of moving the book to production. And I'm indebted to my daughter, Cecilia, for enduring my efforts on this project and offering her suggestions. She's a warm light in my life. And she's a gifted writer who will someday shine a warm light upon the world.

Some of the ideas I set out in this book (and a few of the investigative findings) were first presented in academic and professional journals. Here is a list, in chronological order:

M. Gregg Bloche, "Psychiatry, Capital Punishment, & the Purposes of Medicine," International Journal of Law & Psychiatry 16(3–4) (Summer-Fall 1993) 301–357;

M. Gregg Bloche, "Clinical Loyalties and the Social Purposes of Medicine," Journal of the American Medical Ass'n 281(3) (Jan. 20, 1999) 268–274;

M. Gregg Bloche, "Editorial: Fidelity & Deceit at the Bedside," Journal of the American Medical Ass'n 283(14) (April 12, 2000) 1881–1884;

M. Gregg Bloche & Peter D. Jacobson, "The Supreme Court and Bedside Rationing," Journal of the American Medical Ass'n, 284(21) (Dec. 6, 2000) 2776–2779;

M. Gregg Bloche, "Race & Discretion in American Medicine," Yale Journal of Health Policy, Law, & Ethics 1 (Spring 2001) 95–131;

M. Gregg Bloche, "Caretakers and Collaborators," Cambridge Quarterly of Healthcare Ethics 10(3) (Summer 2001) 275–284;

M. Gregg Bloche, "The Market for Medical Ethics," Journal of Health Policy, Politics, & Law 26(5) (Oct. 2001) 1099–1112;

M. Gregg Bloche, "Trust & Betrayal in the Medical Marketplace," Stanford Law Review 55(3) (Dec. 2002) 919–954;

M. Gregg Bloche, "The Invention of Health Law," California Law Review 91(2) (March 2003) 247–322;

M. Gregg Bloche, "Health Care Disparities—Science, Politics, & Race," New England Journal of Medicine 350(15) (April 8, 2004) 1568–1570;

M. Gregg Bloche, "Back to the '90s—The Supreme Court Immunizes Managed Care," New England Journal of Medicine 351(13) (Sept. 23, 2004) 1277–1279;

M. Gregg Bloche & Jonathan H. Marks, "When Doctors Go to War," New England Journal of Medicine 352(1) (Jan. 6, 2005) 3–6;

M. Gregg Bloche, "American Medicine & the Politics of Race," Perspectives in Biology & Medicine 48(1 Supplement) (Winter 2005) S54–S67;

M. Gregg Bloche, "Obesity & the Struggle Within Ourselves," Georgetown Law Journal 93(4) (April 2005) 1335–1359;

M. Gregg Bloche, "Managing Conflict at the End of Life," New England Journal of Medicine 352(23) (June 9, 2005) 2371–2373;

M. Gregg Bloche & Jonathan H. Marks, "Doctors & Interrogators at Guantanamo Bay," 353(1) (July 7, 2005) 6–8;

M. Gregg Bloche, "The Supreme Court & the Purposes of Medicine," New England Journal of Medicine 354(10) (March 9, 2006) 993–995;

M. Gregg Bloche, "Consumer-Directed Health Care & the Disadvantaged," Health Affairs 26(5) (Sept.-Oct. 2007) 1315–1327;

M. Gregg Bloche, "The Emergent Logic of Health Law," Southern California Law Review 83(3) (March 2009) 389–480.

M. Gregg Bloche
Washington, D.C.
January 2011

chapter one

introduction

hippocrates' myth

Dr. Mara gave my mother her last laugh.[1] Every week or so, Dr. Mara, wearing black, would approach me near the nurses' station to tell me Mom had said, "It's time." At stake were the high-priced bags of blood-clotting cells Dr. Mara reluctantly hung over Mom's bed every few days. The donated cells kept her alive. Leukemia had wiped out her bone marrow, and she couldn't make blood cells. Unless the little straw-colored bags kept appearing atop her intravenous line, she would bleed into her brain, kidneys, and bowels.

Mom's cancer was untreatable. Johns Hopkins had discharged her, and money was a problem. But her dismal prognosis made her eligible for Medicare's hospice benefit. She was a winning financial proposition for any hospice program that would have her—unless the clotting cells were part of the deal. Mom, though, insisted on them. So did I. She was at least as mentally active as I—and determined to astonish her doctors by surviving long past the time they'd given her.

All but one hospice refused to take her unless she agreed to forgo the clotting cells. Transfusions delayed death unnaturally, we were told. They went against hospice thinking about the need to accept the end of life. The program that took her counted on the promise of death within a few weeks.

Weeks, though, stretched into months, and Mom didn't die. Instead, she kept consuming clotting cells and incurring costs that Medicare didn't cover.

Mom stayed alert, without pain, as end-stage leukemia patients often do until their last hours. The first time Dr. Mara told me Mom was "ready" for the treatments to stop, I went into her room girded for the final farewell. But she insisted she'd said no such thing. She begged me to keep the cells coming, which I did. A week later, Dr. Mara, Mom, and I repeated this cycle.

It became a ritual. Mom wouldn't behave like a "good" hospice patient. She wouldn't go without a fight, and Dr. Mara gave her one. Dr. Mara told me the cells were a gift, wasted on my mother since she couldn't be saved. Mom joked about Dr. Mara's black dress and unrelenting efforts to close the Final Sale, until, eventually, leukemia had the Final Say.

Dr. Mara, I suspect, was sincere in her belief that my mother would've been better off without that final fight. She would've taken offense, I'm sure, at the suggestion that money affected either her clinical judgment or her understanding of Mom's wishes. But she also felt that the clotting cells were a precious thing, to be preserved for those who might most benefit from them. I would have seen things her way too, were *my* mother's final hopes not at stake.

I teach and write about health policy. I've cared for patients and advised public officials on what to do about soaring medical costs. During the 2008 presidential campaign, I helped to formulate President Obama's health reform plan. So I'm painfully aware that our medical spending habits are unsustainable. The numbers are scary—the fiscal equivalent of global warming. Within twenty-five years, if we keep on the current track, we'll be spending nearly a third of our income on medical care,[2] unless we learn to say no to pricey treatments that produce tiny benefits.

But don't tell that to me when it's my mother's life that's at stake. And if you're a political office-holder, tell it to the public at your peril. Alarm over "rationing," real or imagined, may well end your career.

As citizens and shoppers, we demand limits on health spending—by voting for politicians who promise to cut taxes and by surfing the web or heading to Wal-Mart to find the lowest prices for products and services. Our pursuit of the best price—for everything from cars, to computers, to lawn care—forces American firms into the breach against medical costs, since more than half of all Americans get their health care coverage through the workplace. But we don't want our doctors to step into the breach alongside the cost-cutters. We expect them to stand with *us* when we're ill and afraid. We expect them to stand by their Hippocratic commitment to their patients, whatever the consequences.

In most medical schools, students make this commitment by reciting the Hippocratic Oath in formal assembly. Some of what they recite hasn't worn well with time. The Oath forbids abortion, rejects surgery, and promises free medical training to its swearers' sons. But the Oath's core premise has stood for more than 2,000 years. "In every house where I come," the Oath proclaims, "I will enter only for the good of my patients."[3] This precept—the doctor's promise to stand for his or her patients without compromise—became a global ideal. It was slow to catch on. The Oath wasn't widely sworn to until centuries after Hippocrates' time.[4] Yet eventually it spread throughout the world, beyond the boundaries of any nation or religion. It was carried west by Roman conquerors, then east by Muslim caliphates. It survived Europe's Dark Ages and the fall and rise of faiths and empires. It became fundamental to the medical profession's conception of itself and to patients' expectations of their doctors. And its core premise—uncompromising commitment to patients—has been embraced by clinical psychologists and others who care for the ill.[5]

Yet this commitment is under unprecedented threat. Medicine's escalating costs and capabilities have transformed it from a politically unnoticed endeavor into a high-profile industry. We can't sustain health care spending that soars to a third or more of our gross domestic product. We'll eventually insist that doctors say no to beneficial or even life-saving treatments because society can't afford them. As I show in this book, physicians are already doing so, covertly. And we'll demand that doctors put their skills and science to use for myriad nontherapeutic purposes—indeed, they already are. Advances in medicine's capabilities are spawning new public applications. Drugs and medical devices are being used to interrogate terror suspects, kill condemned inmates, and enhance performance at school and work, in sports, and in battle. Doctors opine in court and the press on who should be blamed for overeating, smoking, acting on sexual desire, and committing crimes of violence. Medicine, moreover, has become a weapon in our national battles over abortion, same-sex desire, and other social and cultural matters.

How to square this expanding range of social purposes with medicine's 2,000-year-old promise to stand by the sick is the central focus of this book. It won't do, I argue, to reject all uses of medical skill, science, and judgment for nontherapeutic purposes. Medicine's soaring costs have made clinical judgment a public matter, and doctors will need to become wise stewards of limited resources. Leaps in our scientific understanding of mind and body can't be cordoned within the clinical realm; innovators beyond the bedside will inevitably seize on the possibilities. Some of these, I contend, pose grave threats to the profession's trustworthiness in the eyes of patients. Others are putting personal liberty and privacy at growing risk. And medicine's rising power as an arbiter of public morals is usurping the authority of our institutions of self-government.

Medicine's furtherance of social purposes is oftentimes veiled. Doctors ration care covertly, and clinical judgment conceals myriad moral and cultural norms. Beliefs about the proper scope of personal responsibility and the balance between freedom and security shape diagnostic categories and therapeutic recommendations. This book probes for medicine's hidden moral content with an eye toward better understanding of the profession's public and intimate roles.

Conflict among medicine's aims, I argue, animates the health sphere's most bitter moral controversies. Curing and caring are sometimes at odds with each other and often at odds with medicine's public purposes. Stewardship of scarce resources, criminal justice and national security, and support for shared moral beliefs are among these purposes. Struggles over who should receive pricey therapies, whether one or another psychiatric diagnosis should excuse a vicious crime, or whether behaviors scorned by many constitute mental illness reflect tensions among medicine's purposes. Debates over whether doctors should ration care or coach CIA interrogators reflect conflict between public purposes and Hippocratic commitment to patients.

Doctors encounter this conflict within work settings that put pressure on them to go along. Too often, they've gone too far. They've prescribed dubious therapies in response to dubious financial rewards, abetted torture, and covered up clandestine killings. We've countenanced these things, in America and abroad, by tolerating business and political arrangements that invite them. And doctors have rationalized these bad behaviors to themselves as somehow beneficial to patients, required to defeat foreign enemies, or otherwise necessary for the public good. The risk of such rationalization underscores the need to draw lines: to set clear limits on what doctors can do on society's and the state's behalf.

Power and Myth: Medicine's Public Roles

Before Hippocrates, ill health was a sign of divine dismay. The gods had expectations, not always knowable but best not crossed. Diagnosis and treatment demanded an appreciation of their whims and wants. Greek healers who came before Hippocrates were devoted to the supernatural. Asclepius, the Greek god of healing, started out as the mortal son of Apollo. In Homer's *Iliad*, he's both a warrior and a healer. By one account, Asclepius's powers grew to the point that he enraged Hades by reviving the dead, threatening to shrink Hades' domain. Hades conveyed his anger to Zeus, who killed the uppity mortal with a thunderbolt. This, in turn, aroused the wrath of Apollo. Apollo's retribution was quick: he slew the Cyclops, makers of thunderbolts. A chastened Zeus then tried to set things right with Apollo by bringing Asclepius back as a god. Priests of Asclepius were public officials. Ancient sources record their astonishing feats—impregnation of infertile women, restoration of sight to a man with empty eye sockets, removal of spear points from soldiers' lungs, and enabling the lame to walk simply by instructing them to do so. Medicine's therapeutic and social roles were, at the time, without distinction. Cure required pleasing God. It was thus a public matter, no less so than pleas for divine intervention to avert military or natural disaster.

Cities sponsored temples and prescribed rituals. Patients pursued cure by doing their social and religious duty, and priests saw their supplicants' welfare as a by-product of devotion to the gods.

Hippocrates and his followers broke sharply with this way of thinking. They made the radical claim that illness arises from the natural world and that cures thus should be based on the workings of the body. To this end, they put the patient at the center of their endeavors. They collected detailed case histories, rejected religious explanations, and crafted remedies—mainly diet, exercise, and mixed minerals and herbs—based on their physical understandings of sickness.

Hippocrates himself was an unlikely rebel. His family claimed descent from Asclepius himself. The Oath for which he is famed—although he almost certainly didn't write it—opens by invoking Asclepius, Apollo, and other gods as witnesses. But the gods are decorations. Hippocrates focused on illness's mundane, material causes and on the craft of clinical observation. Diet and drugs, not incantations, he claimed, accounted for the priests' treatment successes. In a clever bit of triangulation (it was risky, then as now, to seem dismissive of faith), he said that those who blamed the gods for disease were guilty of blasphemy. The intellectual leaders of classical Athens, including Plato,[6] also gave lip service to the gods, but they embraced Hippocrates's unmagical analytics of clinical classification and cause.

This inward turn, from the demands of the divine to the needs of the body, had momentous implications for the ethics of medicine. It shrank medicine's moral domain, from the social realm to the life of the individual. Hippocrates's followers proclaimed their devotion to the patient as a person, and they set out to win their patients' trust. To this end, they foreswore sex with patients, emphasized accurate prognosis, and avoided curative promises they couldn't keep. They also introduced *privacy* to the doctor-patient relationship. Since the gods neither caused nor cured illness, the personal lives of the sick weren't their business. More to the point, what went on between doctors and patients wasn't the business of priests, politicians, or others who wielded power by claiming to know the gods' will.

The Hippocratic Oath affirms these commitments to the patient. It challenges doctors to resist market pressures, social expectations, and the state's demands. Its promise of loyalty to patients is central to its pledge-taker's professional identity. It has endured for 2,000 years because it appeals powerfully to people's yearnings for someone to stand by them when sickness stirs anxiety and fear. The Hippocratic vow of fidelity, moreover, is therapeutic in itself. A growing body of research shows that patients' belief in their doctors' commitment and competence makes treatment more effective.[7]

But part of what sustained the Hippocratic promise of uncompromising commitment to patients for twenty-some centuries was medical technology's inability to accomplish much. Soldiers, police, and public officials were disinclined to turn to doctors for help in protecting (or oppressing) citizens, since their methods had so little to offer. Medicine could predict the course of illnesses but could do almost nothing to treat them. Its failed remedies were often ghoulish—bloodletting, cutting without anesthesia, and toxic mineral brews. And medicine was cheap to the point of economic irrelevance from a policy perspective. All but the poorest could afford its mostly pointless ministrations; thus those in power had little reason to fret about its cost.

Not until the nineteenth century did this start to change. It can fairly be said that the change began on October 16, 1846, in an operating arena overseen by a dentist, John Warren, at the Massachusetts General Hospital. Warren's guest that day, William Morton, asked a patient to inhale ether before a surgical procedure that would otherwise have been pure agony—slicing into the patient's neck to take out a tumor.[8] The operation was painless and a triumph. Within a few months, pioneering surgeons around the world were using ether to put their patients to sleep—and to open a new universe of therapeutic possibility. Six years later, a British doctor gave chloroform to Queen Victoria for the birth of Prince Leopold.[9] Religious fundamentalists were outraged—scripture enjoined women to bring forth in pain—but popular interest was enormous. Anesthesia quickly became commonplace in operating theaters around the world.

The problem of infection remained. Surgeons operated with dirty instruments, in filthy surroundings, wearing unwashed, blood-splattered frocks. But over the next few decades, the profession grudgingly came to grips with this problem, belatedly acknowledging proof of the germ theory of disease. Surgeons began sterilizing their instruments, first with acid, then with heat. They abandoned their filthy frocks in favor of sterile gowns, and they donned gloves and masks and bathed wounds in antiseptics. The results were astonishing. Deaths from such common procedures as amputation and repair of compound fractures dropped from 50 percent or more to low double digits or less. More than that, the revolutions in anesthesia and antisepsis opened the body to the surgeon's blade. Agonizing pain and deadly putrefaction had kept the chest, abdomen, and brain off-limits; now medicine could invade these biological sancta as a matter of routine.

By the beginning of the twentieth century, X-rays, the electrocardiogram, and a host of other innovations had added to medicine's capabilities and costs. No longer could a doctor deliver state-of-the-art care out of a saddlebag, riding from house to house or town to town. Medicine had begun its march from a nineteenth-century cottage endeavor to an industrial-scale enterprise. Locating anesthesia, antisepsis, and other emerging capabilities in a central setting, typically the hospital, made economic sense. The needed rooms, equipment, and other gadgetry required large numbers of patients to cover their costs. But with rising capabilities came rising public expectations—and rising pressure on governments to make medicine's promise available to all. Germany was the first to do so, offering national health insurance to its citizens in 1883, as a salve for the battlefield sacrifices its leaders demanded in wars against most of its neighbors.[10] Other European nations followed, making medicine a public matter as never before. At the turn of the last century, medical care was a percentage point or less of their economic activity,[11] but the stage was set for state involvement in the setting of priorities and the imposition of limits.

As medicine's capabilities grew—and as expectations soared beyond the profession's ability to deliver—society turned to doctors to perform a broader array of functions that fit awkwardly with the Hippocratic premise of an eye single to patients. Criminal responsibility, once the province of laypeople and priests, became, in the nineteenth and twentieth centuries, a question for physicians. "Madness" became "insanity" (a nineteenth-century clinical term), and "alienists"—so called because the insane were said to be "alienated" from themselves—opined on whether "disease of the mind"[12] kept criminals from controlling their conduct[13] or grasping its wrongfulness.[14] Medicine's dawn-of-the-twentieth-century diagnostic and therapeutic possibilities put doctors front and center in the Great War, as conservators of desperately needed manpower and arbiters of soldiers' fitness to fight. Doctors who judged killers' criminal accountability or soldiers' fitness for combat hardly functioned within the Hippocratic tradition. Their clinical assessments put their "patients" at risk for disastrous consequences—execution (or life in prison) or being maimed or killed on the battlefield.

Dramatic nineteenth-century advances in scientific understanding of contagious disease encouraged another non-Hippocratic possibility: confinement of the sick against their will and compulsory vaccination of the healthy to stop infectious outbreaks. Medicine's grasp of the mechanisms of contagion put public health at odds with fidelity to individuals. Clinical diagnosis could save the lives of those not yet afflicted—if physicians were willing to put the interests of these nonpatients ahead of Hippocratic loyalty.

More subtly, medicine's rising cultural cachet gave it growing influence on public values. Late nineteenth-century physician groups fervently opposed abortion, encouraging popular belief that it constituted the taking of life. Some of the state laws struck down in 1973 by *Roe v. Wade* were inspired by this professional opposition a century earlier. Likewise, nineteenth-century medical thinking both reflected and reinforced the widespread belief that women's mental and physical frailty made them ill-suited for careers in law, business, public affairs—and medicine. All of this, though, was mere prologue for the explosion in medicine's capabilities and costs that has ensued since. Hippocratic purity is no longer possible, if indeed it ever was.

Clinical Care-giving and the Common Good

The Hippocratic promise of uncompromising loyalty to patients has kept us from starting a candid conversation about medicine's expanding public roles. It shames doctors from admitting, even to themselves, that they serve social purposes, sometimes at their patients' expense. And it encourages citizens to expect their doctors to disregard the common good. The result is near-silence about medicine's social uses—and an inability to discuss the drawing of lines between acceptable and intolerable public purposes. Meanwhile, medicine's surging capabilities are increasing the pressure on physicians and other health professionals to break with their promise of fidelity to patients. Soaring costs will compel them to withhold life-extending care to save money. New technologies will seize the interest of governments focused on public security. Political partisans will solicit medical opinion to support myriad claims.

A main purpose of this book is to begin a conversation about how to address medicine's reach into our public life. This conversation needs to engage citizens, not just their doctors. It ought to enlist legislators, judges, military and business leaders, and others who look to medicine with nontherapeutic objectives in mind. It should aim to distinguish between social purposes that are benevolent, or at least bearable, and those that are legally or morally beyond the pale. In the chapters ahead, I report on medicine's rapidly expanding public role. I sound an alarm about the dangers it poses to the profession's credibility as a caring endeavor, to our freedom from the state's intrusion into our intimate lives, and to lay sovereignty over a widening range of moral and social questions. And I argue for restraints that control these dangers while enabling society to take advantage of much that medicine has to offer in the public sphere. The first five chapters that follow this Introduction take up the role of doctors as stewards of scarce resources. I begin in chapters 2 and 3 with a truth that's unmentionable in public life but that's emerging as an existential challenge for our country: Medicine's therapeutic potential is surpassing our ability to pay for it. We can't afford to spend a third of our national wealth on health services a quarter century from now, and we won't: We will ration care. Indeed, we already are, without admitting it. For political leaders, health plan executives, and other keepers of health care resources, the "R-word" is unspeakable. But both public and private health insurers are looking for ways to making spending limits stick. And they're pressing doctors to become their allies in this effort.

Physicians are increasingly going along. They keep mum about some of the pricey possibilities they could offer, and they dissuade us from demanding others on the ground that they're unnecessary. But "medical necessity"—the legal standard for health insurance coverage in the United States and throughout much of the world—is a malleable notion, more of a euphemism for physician habit than a scientific yardstick. And physician habits are shaped by economic influences, including rewards for withholding costly care and penalties for exceeding spending limits. Doctors don't admit this to their patients or even to themselves. The Hippocratic Myth silences them— and stands in the way of a national conversation about how to handle the gap between what medicine might accomplish and what society is willing and able to pay. I offer some ideas about how to manage this gap—how to control medical costs without eviscerating patients' trust. Chapters 4 and 5 probe more deeply, examining the moral and political premises that underlie clinical priority-setting by physicians. Medical judgment, I argue, inescapably incorporates such premises. It reflects and reinforces beliefs about class, race, sex, personal responsibility, and the boundaries between the normal and the nonconforming in human affairs. These beliefs shape spending priorities, definitions of illness, and diagnostic and therapeutic decisions. Their influence is often benign but sometimes pernicious, as when prejudices tied to class or race affect the care people receive.

The Hippocratic tradition fails to acknowledge this. To the contrary, physicians typically claim that their clinical decisions are, or should be, apart from politics. This denial forecloses the possibility of candid conversation about medical judgment's political and moral premises. It shelters prejudice from scrutiny and disempowers patients from making choices about their own bodies based on their own values. It's also dismissive of democratic mechanisms for the setting of health policy priorities. Only by setting aside the myth that medicine is above politics can we begin a searching discussion of the values encrypted within clinical practice. And only by launching such a conversation can we uncover tacit prejudices, empower patients as health decision makers, and ensure that markets and politics, not unaccountable professionals, make the big choices about stewardship of limited medical resources.

In chapter 6, I look at the proposition that doctors who stint on care to save money don't violate their pledge of fidelity to patients so long as patients consent to cost consciousness before the fact. By signing up for health plans that promise to economize, the argument goes, patients declare their *preference* for bedside frugality. They then reap the rewards (lower premiums) and can't later claim betrayal by doctors who don't deliver pricey services provided to those who pay more. It's the choice you make while you're well that counts: You pick a plan, take your chances, and make do with the cards you're dealt. Losers in the lottery of sickness and health might wish they'd signed up for more forgiving coverage, but there are no do-overs—the economics of cost spreading through insurance couldn't work that way. Your *authentic* choice—the one your doctor should honor (this story holds)—is your pick among health plans before you get sick.

Well into the 1980s, this was fringe thinking. Among right-leaning health policy wonks, it's now conventional wisdom. It's the answer HMO advocates give to critics of efforts to coax doctors to withhold costly treatments and keep mum to patients about them. It finesses the problem of conflicting loyalties by denying it. Doctors who limit care on insurers' behalf aren't betraying their patients; they're *honoring* their patients' preferences for frugality. I show why this finesse fails—why the consent that's claimed doesn't extend to a doctor's double agenda as caregiver and naysayer. Popular outrage over this double agenda drove the late 1990s backlash against managed care. This history teaches a powerful lesson: Health reform that relies on betrayal of trust to save money is unsustainable. The gap between medicine's therapeutic potential and our ability to pay for it needs to be faced with a forthrightness that we've so far failed to marshal.

In chapter 7, I turn to medicine's expanding role as an instrument of national security. In the immediate wake of the 9/11 terror attacks, the Bush administration turned to clinical psychologists, psychiatrists, and other physicians to devise interrogation methods that bordered on torture (and in the view of many, crossed that border). Doctors designed these methods, oversaw their use, and were central to the administration's efforts to legally justify them. I tell this story with an eye toward its larger lessons about what can go wrong when doctors become warriors, unmoored from Hippocratic ideals. Parts of the story are known from journalistic accounts. I report other parts here for the first time, based on interviews with principals who haven't previously spoken publicly, as well as on documents newly obtained. And I spotlight other, emerging uses of medicine for military purposes. Some could make military action more humane and effective; others promise to make it more barbaric.

Chapter 8 considers professional leaders' sleight-of-hand response to revelations that doctors had critical roles in post-9/11 detainee abuse. The organizations that represent American psychologists and psychiatrists claimed fealty to Hippocratic ideals but countenanced conduct that flagrantly breached them. Participants in the planning of harsh interrogations played a pivotal role in crafting ethics loopholes that protected their own from prosecution and professional sanctions. An opportunity to set clear limits on use of clinical skills and judgment for national security purposes was thereby lost. I conclude this chapter by proposing some limits—limits that preserve patient trust (and personal rights) while recognizing biomedical science's potential to protect us from foreign foes.

In chapter 9, I examine the law's growing reliance on clinical judgment. Courts and legislators have increasingly turned to medicine to make choices that lie beyond the scope of doctors' expertise. Over the last hundred years, psychiatrists became central to the ascription of criminal responsibility. More recently, physicians and psychologists have become key decision makers when divorcing spouses battle over child custody. They're emerging as gatekeepers to drugs that boost academic performance. And both liberals and conservatives look to doctors to take their side in struggles over abortion, obesity, and other matters at the interface between biology and politics. It's hardly surprising that doctors aren't of one mind about such matters, but

it's dismaying that they haven't shown more restraint. Medical pronounce-
ments on these questions bootstrap on cultural and moral premises. Not
only is bootstrapping of this sort disingenuous; it undermines confidence
in physicians' commitment to patients by spending professional credibility
to promote bitterly contested claims. Chapter 9 also looks at use of medical
technologies to achieve the law's purposes. At times, judges conform these
uses to Hippocratic ideals (the Supreme Court allowed doctors to opt out of
lethal injection); more often, courts utterly ignore these ideals.

I conclude in chapter 10 with some overarching ideas about accommodation between medicine's caregiving and public roles. Realistic accommodation must begin with recognition that we burden our doctors with contradictory expectations. Like my mother, we want them to stand by us without
compromise, especially in desperate times. But this longing is at odds with
our thinking about the common good. We *want* physicians to control runaway medical costs, to protect us from peril, and to share and affirm our ideals. By failing to acknowledge medicine's public purposes, the Hippocratic
Oath denies the need to consider what doctors should do—and what we
should expect from them—when public and private purposes conflict.

What's needed is a national (indeed global) conversation about the permissible ends of medicine—a conversation that ends the silence about social purposes that the Oath imposes. The primacy of medicine's caring role
should be the starting point for this conversation. Trust engendered in clinical relationships shouldn't be violated. Doctors shouldn't withhold beneficial
care to save money, absent candor and clarity about the cost-benefit balances
being struck. They shouldn't use their clinical skills to kill on the state's behalf, either as warriors or executioners, even when it's acceptable for others to
do these things. But medical practice can and should take public values into
account. Clinical practice guidelines that count cost are a policy imperative
if America is to avert fiscal catastrophe. And medical judgments that incorporate widely shared values are part of our cultural fabric. Cost-benefit trade-
offs and moral premises that undergird clinical judgment, though, should be
open to public discussion and decision. It won't do to put them off-limits,
as both liberals and conservatives are wont to do, by insisting that medical

practice stay apart from economics and politics. Beyond the clinical realm, we should encourage doctors to put their skills to use for the common good. But they should do so in ways that neither breach trust built in clinical relationships nor misportray moral preferences as scientific conclusions.

In the years ahead, medicine's place in our public life will grow as its costs and capabilities soar. Advances in the brain sciences, genomics, and other areas will give doctors new powers to explain, intervene, absolve, and destroy. Government and private actors will be tempted to use these powers for their own purposes, and physicians will be tempted (or pressed) to go along. There is thus a critical need to define the permissible ends of medicine. This book represents a beginning.

chapter two

cutting costs
and keeping faith

Carrie

Every few months or so, since her mid-teens, Carrie Emard became con-vinced that she was about to die. "You know when it's going to hit," she told me. "Your stomach just starts giving you warning signals—it just starts hurting and starts bloating. You feel you need to go, but you can't—your body doesn't let you, and you start shaking."[1]

Several times, her husband came home to find Carrie on the bathroom floor, sweating and moaning, feeling like she'd been stabbed. One October night in 2005, her husband lay on top of her, then held her, to try to stop the shaking. The next thing she remembers of the episode is humiliation as firemen and paramedics carried her outside, wearing only a bra. "I'm embar-rassed and feeling like I'm crazy. The chief of firemen and paramedics was a friend. At least he stayed outside and looked the other way." On the way to the hospital, her pain subsided. The doctors scolded her for calling an ambulance. "It was like, you weren't really that bad—you weren't really that sick—you're kind of crazy."

Carrie's symptoms were an enigma to her doctors but not to her. A doz-en years earlier, at age eleven, she'd had her first period. It was painful and heavy, like all her periods since. By age thirteen, she was missing school a day or two each month. Her mother took her to a doctor, who said it was just cramps. A year later, she went on the pill to control her periods, but this didn't stop the pain. Then, maybe a few months later, Carrie's mom came home one night and collapsed. "We got her up," Carrie recalls, "and she said, 'I'm okay.'" But that's when Carrie learned that her mother had endured pain like Carrie's for many years.

Her mother's monthly pains remained a mystery. "She grew up in a poor family—she was one of seven kids." She didn't think of seeing a doctor. "Her attitude was, 'You have bad cramps, and you just have to move on and just don't let it mess up your life.'" Then, soon after Carrie turned fifteen, her mom had a spasm of pain like no other. "She went to the emergency room," Carrie remembers, "and the surgeons opened her up." Bloody tufts of uterine tissue were growing all over her pelvis. "It was everywhere," Carrie told me, "from her ovaries to her colon."

Carrie's mother had an especially bad case of endometriosis, so-called because the growths look and act like uterine lining.[2] They enlarge early in the menstrual cycle, then bleed when women get their periods. It's this bleeding that causes the pain. The stray clumps of uterine tissue "menstruate" into a woman's body—into her abdomen instead of out through her vagina. Once-a-month agony is a common result. So Carrie became convinced she had what her mom had—severe endometriosis, unrecognized by her doctors.

Doctors call endometriosis a "surgical diagnosis"—a euphemism for a diagnosis you can make only by cutting into a patient to take a look. But Carrie's doctors didn't want to operate—not after trials of birth control pills failed, not after her 2005 ER visit, not after follow-on episodes of pain so bad that she imagined death as a relief. She tried herbal concoctions and quirky diets, to no avail; then she switched health plans and sought out a doctor for surgery. An operating room date was scheduled, then chance intervened: In August 2006, Carrie learned she was pregnant.

Her unplanned pregnancy had an unplanned effect—her symptoms disappeared. "While I was pregnant," she told me years later, "I felt better than I ever felt before." Carrie looked forward to becoming a mom. She didn't fret when, on a Saturday in late September, she saw blood seeping out of her vagina. The rep on the other end of her HMO's advice line did fret, telling her to go to the hospital to check it out. In the ER, the blood flowed faster. Carrie remembers bits and pieces of what happened next—some cramps, an ultrasound, then a rushed prep for surgery. The on-call gynecologist, Dr. Claire Leve, told her that the embryo had taken root in her left fallopian tube, not her uterus, and that there was a one in three chance she would die.

"I started crying. I remember telling my husband, 'Call my mom, call my family, and have them pray for me.' A lot of visitors and my family were there when I woke up from the surgery. I just remember visitors and being in a lot of pain."

The operation turned out to be a mistake—there was no embryo in Carrie's fallopian tube.[3] Removing the tube accomplished nothing—except to make a future pregnancy less likely. Carrie's bleeding, it turned out, was due to a miscarriage—a heartbreaking event, but a common one, occurring in up to 30 percent of all pregnancies.[4] And, Dr. Leve told her as the anesthesia wore off and the pain from her incision set in, there was one other surprise.

Leve showed her photos of her insides—her bowels and other organs—taken during surgery. Little dots, darkish things, were everywhere, it seemed, and they were probably ovarian cancer, catastrophically advanced. Carrie's family prayed, cried, and prepared to take her home. Then the pathology report came in—endometriosis all over. But no cancer, and no death sentence. Just a garden-variety miscarriage—and an unnecessary operation—with endometriosis as an incidental finding. Carrie might have sued for medical malpractice since her pointless surgery made it more probable that she'd never have a child.

Yet Carrie implored Dr. Leve to take her on as a patient. The doctor was a *witness*. She knew Carrie's endometriosis was real. "I felt like I needed Dr. Leve because she'd seen it—she was inside me—and she knew that I wasn't crazy." Leve declined, spooked, Carrie figures, by the mistakenly removed fallopian tube and the possibility of a lawsuit, something Carrie didn't intend. So Carrie went back to her HMO gynecologist, who proposed to put her back on the Pill, which she was sure wouldn't work.

That's when Carrie went way out of line, as her HMO, HealthNet, saw things. Carrie's mom found a surgeon in Oregon, Dr. David Redwine, with an unconventional theory and an unusual approach. A bit of background helps to understand the battle that ensued. Medical students learn that endometriosis happens when women menstruate backward, through their fallopian tubes and into their abdominal cavities.[5] Cells from the uterus, this story holds, take root like crabgrass on the ovaries, bowels, and other internal organs. Because these organs are constantly being "seeded" from the uterus, this story holds, removal of the rogue growths can't cure the disease. Surgeons can weed the garden, but they can't stop the weeds from coming back, since the uterus keeps sowing seeds.

So painstakingly perfect excision of each growth is pointless, according to the standard story. It makes more sense—and costs less money—to manage the pain with pills and to trim back the weeds from time to time through simpler operations when the pain gets out of control. Budget-conscious health plans like this approach, but it consigns women to a lifetime of more or less chronic pain. And the theory behind it has never been proven: Like so much in medicine, the backwards menstruation story is something doctors take on faith.[6]

A much less fashionable theory holds that miscreant stem cells give rise to growths, outside the uterus, of cells that resemble endometrium. These misbehaving cells don't migrate, this story holds; they sit, immobile, in the abdomen, sprouting thickets of disease. These cells remain the stuff of myth—they've never been seen. But Redwine and scattered colleagues elsewhere have embraced this theory and its implication—that endometriosis can be *cured,* once and for all, by cutting out *all* the weeds—the thickets of disease and their unseen stem-cell roots. They point to their own long-term follow-up studies, which health plans have disregarded. Most of the patients they've operated on with cure in mind, these studies have found, stay symptom-free thereafter.[7] This couldn't happen, they contend, if backwards menstruation kept seeding new growths.

These results, they say, justify the approach that health plans don't want to pay for—painstaking (and pricey) surgery to remove every last disease trace. Carrie's HMO gynecologist wanted her to stick to convention—medications to manage her pain, plus periodic, simpler procedures to trim back her growths. But she dreaded the prospect of pain for a lifetime, pain that was threatening her marriage. So she pressed her primary care physician for a referral to Redwine, a referral that would cost her health plan tens of thousands of dollars if she had the surgery Redwine's approach envisioned.

What she didn't know was that the plan penalized doctors who make out-of-plan referrals, docking their pay and giving them lower ratings for performance.[8] Its medical director, moreover, often disallowed such referrals. Her primary care doctor, Jennifer Hopper, tried at first to coax Carrie to go the conventional route. But Carrie came in with printouts of Redwine's articles and other materials she'd found online. She pled her case passionately, and Dr. Hopper came around. "I had a twenty-five-year-old who was looking at multiple laparoscopic procedures over the course of her lifetime versus one definitive procedure," Hopper recalled more than a year later.[9] "She was in a great deal of pain and concerned with fertility. I wanted her out of pain. It was worth a try."

The plan's medical director, Jose Arevelo, decided otherwise. In April 2007, he rejected the referral. Carrie's appeals to HealthNet's management were unsuccessful. Meanwhile, her monthly episodes of anguishing pain continued. And her marriage was unraveling.

From the health plan's perspective, the matter was simple. The studies that supposedly supported Dr. Redwine's unconventional, costly approach had appeared in lesser journals and were of dubious quality. They came nowhere near to medicine's "gold standard" for proof of efficacy—the random sorting of similar patients into groups who receive different therapies, followed by the tracking of clinical outcome measures chosen in advance. All that Redwine and the others had done was to report on the patients *they'd* picked to treat. They'd neither compared their approach to conventional treatments nor chosen their outcome measures in advance. Their results were thus infected with investigator bias (potentially affecting both patient selection and assessment of success) and ill-suited for rendering judgment about the value of Redwine's approach.

Missing from this picture is the awkward truth that much the same could be said of conventional therapies. Birth control pills, other hormonal treatments, and periodic surgeries to destroy easily seen growths haven't been assessed by this gold standard, let alone compared to Redwine's approach. Uncertainty thus suffuses the treatment of endometriosis—uncertainty that doctors rarely share with their patients, since doctors tend to believe passionately that what they do is right.

This mix of uncertainty, competing approaches, and deep conviction is combustible—and much more common in medicine than most patients realize. Professional rivalries and passions stand in the way of reasoned discussion of questions that haven't yet been answered scientifically. Redwine's conviction came from a lifetime of experience excising endometriosis with cutting tools instead of burning it with electrodes or lasers, as gynecologists typically do. "You use your sight and your sense of touch," he told me. "Endometriosis has a feel. It's hard. It can invade deeply—two or three centimeters deep, into bowels and other tissues. Since the laser surgeon isn't dissecting things out, he doesn't know how deeply to go." A laser, he said, "vaporizes only the thickness of a human hair. It's like trying to take out a walnut with a ball point pen"—without being able to feel the walnut. "You need to burn deeply, but you don't know how deeply to burn—you can't burn too deeply without damaging vital structures."

"That's why the world's outstanding laser surgeons can't eliminate endometriosis," Redwine insisted. That's why it recurs. The backward menstruation myth, he argued, is frayed cover for this failing. And the relief experienced by hundreds of patients whom Redwine had treated over the years was powerful proof, for him, that his approach *worked,* whatever health insurers' claims to the contrary.

So Arevelo's refusal to approve the referral was at odds with what Redwine *knew,* from sight, feel, and his patients' gratitude. For centuries, medical knowledge has accrued this way, and despite the explosion of biomedical research over the past century, it still does. The maxim that medicine "is an art, not a science" conveys this truth. But different doctors' lifetimes of experience often yield rival truths about what does and doesn't work. Gynecologists who've mastered the art of the laser tend to "know" that backward menstruation causes endometriosis to recur, that repeat operations are therefore inevitable, and that the simplicity of laser surgery (done through a thin tube, pushed through a tiny incision) minimizes discomfort and risk.

"Medical Necessity"

Medicine has not yet found a way to deal with its rival truths. Over the past several decades, researchers who study the effectiveness of tests and treatments have shown that myriad, widely used therapies don't work—or, even worse, cause more harm than good.[10] Recent, high-profile examples include estrogen replacement therapy for post-menopausal women (meant to reduce their risk of cardiovascular disease) and placement of stents in clogged coronary arteries to prop them open. Giving estrogen to post-menopausal women, it turned out, makes heart attacks and strokes *more* likely.[11] So does putting stents into clogged coronaries.[12] But most of what doctors do has not been put to the empirical test. Wide variations in clinical practice are more the rule than the exception.

So Dr. Arevelo had grounds for treating the Redwine referral as unnecessary—if, by "necessary," one means a sure thing. And since few things are certain in medicine, requiring clear proof of a pricey treatment's superiority is a way to save lots of money. Were health plans to pay only for therapies proven beyond a doubt, most of what doctors do would go uncovered. That would be no loss (except to doctors) if lack of certainty meant no therapeutic benefit. But it doesn't: Uncertainty means there's a possibility of benefit—a possibility forgone when health plans refuse to pay.

That's how health plans ration care, routinely, without admitting it. They almost never refuse to cover care that's a sure thing.[13] But doctors have wide space to ration covertly, under the clouds of scientific doubt. The U.S. Supreme Court has said as much. In June 2000, the justices said federal law allows health plans to reward doctors for withholding beneficial care to save money.[14] A lower court had concluded otherwise, declaring that doing so tramples on the medical profession's "most sacred values"[15] by enticing them to break faith with their patients. Most patients, I daresay, would agree. When I told Carrie that her health plan paid doctors extra for withholding referrals, she voiced shock. "That's insane. It's disgusting. It's a horrible system," she said. "Normal people like me—they don't realize that these things are taking place." But the Supreme Court said rewards for saying no are critical to HMO design. "[W]hatever the HMO," Justice David Souter wrote for the court, "there must be rationing and the inducement to ration. . . . [N]o HMO organization could survive without some incentive connecting physician reward with treatment rationing."[16]

Souter's pronouncement came nine years after Cynthia Herdrich went to her doctor, Lori Pegram, complaining of pain in her groin. Pegram examined her patient and, with her hands, found a swollen, tender area roughly where Herdrich's appendix ought to be. An ultrasound was called for, Pegram decided, and one was available immediately at a local hospital. But the hospital wasn't part of Herdrich's HMO, the Carle Clinic (which rewarded Pegram, a co-owner, for clinical frugality). So Pegram made Herdrich wait more than a week, for a time slot at a Carle Clinic facility fifty miles away. Meanwhile, her appendix ruptured, dumping its infected contents into her abdomen—a life-threatening event. She'd had appendicitis, it turned out, readily treatable with minor surgery if identified in time.

Cynthia Herdrich survived and sued her health plan for importuning Dr. Pegram to stint on care.[17] When I spoke to Cynthia at the Supreme Court on the day her case was argued, she expressed the same sense of violation Carrie would later voice over money paid to doctors to say no. But the court refused to acknowledge her concern.[18] The justices treated such payments as a sort of volume control—a way to dial up and down on clinical cost in pursuit of "optimal treatment levels."[19] And the contract language that governs health insurers' coverage decisions leaves wide space for insurers to dial down on cost—and up on health risks. Almost without exception, insurers promise to pay for care that's "medically necessary," a promise that patients typically understand as a commitment to cover all care that's more likely to do benefit than harm. But this content-free standard does little to cabin clinical nay-saying. It defers to doctors to say what's needed (at least, that's how courts have construed the term), but it permits insurers to pick and choose from among medical opinions.

That's what Dr. Arevelo did: He went with the approach that seemed cheaper, at least in the near term. He cast aside the *chance* that Dr. Redwine's aggressive approach would cure Carrie, and by so doing, he broke faith with her expectation that her doctors would do all they could to help her. Keeping faith with this expectation, though, would bust the budget. Justice Souter underscored this when he spoke the unspeakable, by saying (repeatedly!) that HMOs ration care. And what's true of HMOs is true (albeit with looser constraints) for all the other health plans to which Americans subscribe. *No* plan can afford to cover all the care that *might* be of benefit—all the tests and treatments that flawed studies and physicians' subjective impressions suggest would do more good than harm. Sure, some of these services are, in fact, pointless or harmful: Estrogen replacement and cardiac stents (for most patients) are illustrative. But many yield benefits that arguably outweigh their risks, especially if the benefits that count include hope and a sense of well-being, not just years of life added.

Neither health plans nor politicians want to admit this. The standard story—the *only* story—pushed by plan executives and political office-seekers is that we can control costs by eliminating pure waste—care that yields no benefit or does more harm than good. No insurer advertises, on the sides of buses, that it cuts costs by denying care that extends life at too high a price. And no politician promises to stave off fiscal ruin by rationing Medicare. Through the 2008 presidential campaign, John McCain and Barack Obama spoke of controlling medical costs by encouraging competition, preventing sickness, and cutting waste. The "R-word" was off-limits (as it was in previous campaigns), except as an epithet for the *other* side's health plan. Those who spoke for the campaigns were told to avoid it in favor of scenarios that promised cost control without health consequences.

That withholding beneficial care to control costs is a radioactive proposition in American politics was underscored by the panic over "death panels" and "rationing boards"[20] in 2009, during the run-up to health care reform. Democrats proposed nothing of the kind, but that didn't seem to matter; right-wing pundits played on fears of Hippocratic violation, suborned by government. "Tea Party" opposition to reform—by some accounts a major factor in the Republican Party's 2010 electoral success—was animated by the specter of doctors stinting on care to save money.[21]

As an Obama health policy "surrogate" in 2008, I was told to point out that 30 percent of what we spend on medical care yields no benefit.[22] True—but there's a twist: We don't know, until after the fact, *which* care is pointless *under what conditions*. And we can't quickly find out. A large-scale program of research into the effectiveness of tests and treatments in common use is much needed.[23] But the astonishing variability of patients' responses to care makes case-by-case uncertainty inevitable,[24] and the cumbersome work of studying medical outcomes will always lag behind the explosive pace of clinical innovation. So the 30 percent figure is like the shimmering in the distance on a dessert highway—a goal that perpetually recedes. We can make large cuts in the care that's useless only by curtailing care that saves and improves lives, since we're not able, in most cases, to distinguish between the two.

Health plans make such cuts covertly, under cover of the contractual euphemism, "medical necessity." That's what Carrie's HMO did when it refused to cover Dr. Redwine's potentially curative course of treatment. But Carrie refused to abide by her health plan's verdict. She appealed the denial—first, by making her case to plan bureaucrats, then, when this failed, by invoking a California statute that empowers patients to demand independent physician review of coverage denials. She also took a terrifying risk. Instead of waiting out the appeals process, she flew to Oregon for surgery, putting herself and her husband at risk for bankruptcy if her health plan prevailed. At 9:15 AM on May 3, 2007, Dr. Redwine's surgical team opened Carrie's abdomen to begin the radical procedure he'd prescribed. What he found astonished him. The dark blotches, reddish and brownish, were everywhere, growing out of her reproductive organs and embedded in her bowels. They'd penetrated her diaphragm, invading her chest and inflaming her lungs. Her endometriosis, he recalled, was the worst he'd ever seen.

He set about excising it, slowly, painstakingly. He carved, scraped, and plucked the small growths from her liver, spleen, stomach, and gut. Fearing that he'd penetrate her bowels fully, he removed several feet of intestines, hoping to avoid catastrophic post-op infection. His team extended their incision into her chest, looking to keep her disease from taking sanctuary near her lungs. They operated for more than nine hours, and when it was over, Redwine felt confident he'd gotten everything.

But the extensive dissection of Carrie's abdomen left massive scarring, scarring that stiffened and constricted some organs and caused others to attach to her abdominal walls. Over the next three months, she endured a series of life-threatening complications. Carrie suffered mysterious, spiking fevers and returned to the operating room multiple times—for a collapsed lung, several bowel blockages, and a gallbladder that stopped working. All the while, she battled her HMO, which refused to pay as her bills mounted.

On July 26, five days after surgery to remove her gallbladder, she went for a routine follow-up appointment with Dr. Jadaborg, one of Redwine's associates. Carrie's blood pressure was dangerously low, and her heart rate was worrisomely high, signs of severe dehydration. Dr. Jadaborg started an intravenous line and gave her two liters (about a half-gallon) of fluid. The next day, Carrie came back for another two liters of IV fluids. Her heart rate and blood pressure normalized. She experienced no further worrisome symptoms. More than a year later, she was still without complications. The monthly episodes of agony that had afflicted her since age thirteen never returned. Cure, or something resembling it, had been achieved—at a cost that reached $250,000.

On June 15, 2007, Carrie's HMO, HealthNet, told her it had rejected her appeal on the ground that "surgery for endometriosis could have been provided within the medical group network" to which HealthNet had assigned her—the network on whose behalf Dr. Arevelo had said no. Since no one within this network offered the procedure she'd received, the unspoken but unmistakable message was that the plan would pay only for the conventional approach. "The fact that a physician . . . may perform [or] prescribe" a service, HealthNet said in its denial letter, "does not, in itself, make it medically necessary."

But HealthNet had overreached. Its definition of "medical necessity" (a definition that was part of its contract with Carrie) required it to provide coverage, regardless of cost, when there is "credible scientific evidence" of a treatment's superiority.[25] This gave Carrie an opening, and she seized it. With help from Redwine, she wrote to California's Department of Managed Health Care, demanding independent medical review of HealthNet's refusal to pay.[26] She marshaled the less-than-perfect scientific evidence Redwine had assembled, including flawed studies published in second-line journals, suggesting his approach yielded superior outcomes. She couldn't prove her case beyond a doubt—the studies' methodological defects[27] left lots of room for quibbling. But all she needed to do was to persuade the reviewers that Redwine's approach was more likely than not to give her better results.

On October 30, 2007, word came that she had done so. The firm retained by California's Department of Managed Health Care to conduct independent reviews told her it was overturning HealthNet's denial of coverage on the ground that Redwine's approach was "medically necessary." HealthNet tried to cut its losses by refusing to pay for the follow-up care occasioned by Carrie's difficult post-op course. But Carrie battled back, disputing these denials and eventually persuading HealthNet that further niggling would be futile. By August 2008, HealthNet had agreed to pay every last outstanding bill. Carrie had been symptom-free for more than a year. Her doctors told her to count herself as cured. But the physical agonies, financial terrors, and embittering struggles with her HMO were too much for her marriage. She'd filed for divorce the previous September, just weeks before winning her appeal. The divorce was finalized in April. After her doctors cleared her, she headed off in October to Peru, to spend the next year, or maybe more, working with orphaned kids. "Life is good," she told me before she left. "I'm excited to be alive."

Carrie eluded Dr. Arevelo's and HealthNet's limit-setting efforts by dint of her persistence and uncommon courage. She caught HealthNet in the maw of its own contradiction—its unwillingness to openly countenance rationing and its effort to economize by refusing to cover potentially beneficial care. Dr. Arevelo embodied this contradiction. As medical director of the physician network to which Carrie was assigned, he had to work within a budget. HealthNet paid the network a flat, per-patient fee each year; out of this pool of money, the network had to cover all of its HealthNet patients' costs. So Averelo had to ration care to keep within budget. But he couldn't admit to doing so, since HealthNet's contractual definition of "medical necessity" forbade the counting of costs against clinical benefits. This definition opened the way for Carrie to take her case beyond Averelo—to call *HealthNet* on its failure to cover Redwine's radical, costly, and promising therapy.

Carrie had formidable resources—smarts, savvy, steely resolve, and laws that empowered her to push back when her plan said no. For patients without these means—and for physicians who face wide gaps between what patients expect and resources permit—the Hippocratic ideal of uncompromising commitment to the patient is more elusive.

Yanira

The Hippocratic ideal was out of reach for Yanira Montanez, who lived in one of the roughest parts of Philadelphia with her mother Iris, her twelve-year-old brother, and her four-month-old daughter. On a Friday evening in March 2004, Yanira, who'd just turned twenty, came down with a headache. She tried Tylenol, then fell asleep, but when she woke early in the morning, the headache was worse. She took some more Tylenol, then some Motrin, but the headache wouldn't go away. Iris helped her with the baby, and she got some sleep on Saturday and Sunday nights. On Monday, Iris woke at 6, then fed her granddaughter. But by 7, Iris was out the door—off to the second day of a two-week welfare-to-work training program. Alone with her baby, Yanira became afraid. And she began to experience weakness in her right arm, and trouble grasping things with the fingers in her right hand.

"When I came home from work," Iris recalled in an interview four years later, "she told me she couldn't pick up the baby's toy—she dropped it in the baby's face." Yanira's face and lips went numb, she couldn't eat or drink, and that night she began throwing up. By Tuesday morning, she had right leg weakness as well. At Iris's urging, she called her doctor. A nurse took the call, asked Yanira about her symptoms, then told her to phone 911. Iris desperately wanted to go to the hospital with her daughter, but that would have meant being a no-show for job training. Being a no-show would have meant the end of Iris's welfare payments, on which the family depended.

So Yanira went alone, by ambulance, to the emergency room, after arranging for the baby's father—her on-again, off-again fiancé—to care for their daughter. Yanira's twelve-year-old brother, Wilson, stayed home from school, then walked a half mile to the hospital by himself to be with her. Yanira arrived at Temple University's Episcopal Hospital at about 10:15 that morning and waited about an hour for an emergency room triage nurse. Hospital records show she told the nurse she "couldn't keep anything down" and had headaches and numbness in her right hand. But when an ER doctor saw her, he ordered no diagnostic tests. Records show he performed only a cursory physical exam, gave her a drug that speeds stomach contractions, then sent her home with some Tylenol. All in all, he spent only a few minutes with her. His "diagnosis": "Nausea/Vomiting," a restatement of her chief complaint.

By 1 PM, Yanira was back home, having walked by shuffling sideways, at times clinging to Wilson for support. For a time, the stomach medicine seemed to work, easing her nausea and enabling her to get some sleep. She dozed intermittently through the afternoon and into the night, but she woke the next morning with a severe headache, worsening facial numbness, and renewed vomiting. Again, Yanira called her doctor and was told by a nurse to go to the emergency room. And again, her mother Iris faced a Dickensian dilemma: Should she take her daughter to the ER (and fail to show for job training), or should she leave Yanira to fend for herself—alone, afraid, and at grave risk?

Getting cut off from welfare wasn't an option. So Iris went to training. Wilson went to school. And instead of braving the ER alone, Yanira stayed home. As the day wore on, her symptoms grew worse. Her right arm became weaker, and she continued to vomit. When her mom came home from training, they went to the hospital—a different hospital this time, farther from home, since the doctor at Episcopal hadn't helped. Yanira and Iris arrived at Northeastern Hospital's crowded emergency room at about 5:30 PM, then waited until after 9 to be seen by a doctor. Again, Yanira told the ER staff about her headaches, nausea and vomiting, arm weakness, and numbness. And again the doctor rushed through an exam, failing to pursue her complaints of headache, weakness, and numbness by doing a detailed neurologic assessment. According to Iris, he spent "maybe three minutes" talking to and examining Yanira.

This time, at least, the doctor ordered a few lab studies, including a pregnancy test, which came back positive. He attributed her nausea and vomiting to early pregnancy, ascribed her headache to "hyperventilation," gave her some prenatal vitamins, and sent her home. "I asked, if she's pregnant, why all this right-side numbness, weakness," Iris recalls. He didn't reply. By midnight, Yanira was home. She lay down, slept, then woke the next day with the same symptoms. Her mother gave her a talking-to for getting pregnant. "I said, 'Your baby's four months old, and now you're pregnant again. You're stuck with another baby now.'" "Abortion," she told me, "we really don't believe in that."

Iris then left home for her next-to-last day of job training. Through the course of the day, Yanira's headache, vomiting, and weakness became worse. Shortly before midnight, she decided to return to Northeastern Hospital, this time accompanied by her fiancé. She waited more than five hours to see a doctor, who drew another blood test for pregnancy and gave her some worrisome news: the level of the hormone that showed she was pregnant had *dropped* slightly over the past day, from 5823 to 5315.[28] Because this hormone, beta hCG, is produced by the placenta (it's not made by women who aren't pregnant), it typically *rises* rapidly as pregnancy progresses and the placenta grows, doubling in concentration every two to three days during the early weeks. So something was amiss, and the ER doctor, Robert Davies, took a low-cost step to explore it, ordering a pelvic ultrasound to assess the status of Yanira's pregnancy.

The results were puzzling. An ultrasound offers a glimpse into the womb, in the form of reflections from sound waves sent into the uterus. Dr. Davies saw something in Yanira's womb—a fluid-filled, cyst-like space. But there was neither a yolk sac nor a heartbeat—things he figured he'd see in a pregnancy far enough along to produce a beta hCG of more than 5000. "I definitely expected to see evidence of a pregnancy," he later recalled. "I saw evidence of a pregnancy [but] did not see evidence of a fetus."

He might, at this point, have pursued the question further, by ordering a more sophisticated scan, perhaps an MRI. But in the early morning hours, in an ER overstretched by the vast, unmet needs of one of America's most blighted urban areas, such pursuit wasn't in the cards. There was a crush of patients still to be seen. And the mismatch between urgent clinical needs and the hospital's high-tech resources raised the threshold for tapping these resources. So Dr. Davies relied on the limited facts he had and made the most plausible inference—that Yanira was probably having a miscarriage.

The hospital record indicates that Davies thought Yanira was still pregnant—and told her so. Davies later insisted that he thought, but wasn't certain, that the pregnancy was in the process of aborting. In any event, he sent Yanira home at about 6 AM, with an antibiotic for a minor urinary infection and instructions to see her gynecologist a few days later. "It's really a little premature to say that the pregnancy was definitely going to end in miscarriage," he argued years later, defending his decision. "We really have to do that over more time. Usually, we repeat the beta [hCG] roughly a week later, and see that there's a more significant decline. . . . And if there isn't a decline, probably an ultrasound would be repeated."

A few minutes after Yanira got home, her mother left for the last day of welfare-to-work training. Yanira went to sleep—it's uncertain for how long. Six hours later, just after noon, she fell down a flight of thirteen steps. How this happened isn't known. It's unclear whether she first lost consciousness, or whether she merely tripped or lost her balance. What's certain is that she was found unresponsive at the bottom of the stairs, then taken to Temple University Hospital by ambulance. At Temple, she remained unresponsive to all efforts to rouse her. Doctors intubated her, then sent her for a head CT scan, a test no one had ordered during her three earlier ER visits.

The scan's multiple cross-sections of the brain revealed an unfolding catastrophe. A large mass of tissue, almost certainly a tumor, was growing on the left side, pushing her normal, jelly-like brain tissue downward. The pressure created by the mass had forced part of her brain out through the fora-men magnum, an opening at the base of the skull through which the spinal column rises to meet the brainstem. Arteries that carry oxygen to much of the brain were squeezed shut by the downward shift. A follow-up MRI scan confirmed the dismal picture. Yanira had almost certainly suffered devastat-ing injury to the centers of thought, feelings, and muscle movement. And she was at imminent risk of dying—unless the pressure in her skull from the expanding mass and the trauma could somehow be relieved.

Iris learned of her daughter's fall, but not its seriousness, when she called home. High doses of steroids, given intravenously, were doing little to lower the pressure. Repeated scans showed ongoing brain displacement and rising danger. When Iris finally saw her daughter, in the early evening, she was un-responsive to voice, touch, and even pain. Through the night, Yanira's neuro-logical status declined. The next morning, one of her doctors called Iris and asked her to make a terrible decision: "He said they needed to do emergency surgery and if they didn't do the surgery, my daughter wasn't going to make it for more than maybe an hour, maybe two." The surgeons proposed to open Yanira's skull and to cut away at least some of the mystery mass. This would reduce the rising pressure. It would give the doctors a fighting chance to save Yanira's life. But it posed enormous risks. It could kill her immediately, and it could destroy parts of the brain that shape personality, thought, perception, and movement.

Iris consented to the surgery on Yanira's behalf. The operation lasted eight hours. When it was over, a massive tumor had been mostly removed from the left side of her brain. Pathology studies of slides from the tumor confirmed that it was cancerous. But it wasn't a brain tumor, or, at least, it didn't start out as one. It was choriocarcinoma—a rare cancer that forms in the womb from placental tissue gone awry. It explained the odd findings on the ultrasound a few days before—the evidence of pregnancy without evi-dence of a fetus—and it explained Yanira's positive blood test for pregnancy. Doctors treat the hormone beta hCG as diagnostic of pregnancy because the placenta makes it. But so does cancer of the placenta. Follow-on studies con-firmed that Yanira had advanced choriocarcinoma. The tumor had begun in her uterus, just after her pregnancy, then spread through her blood to her brain and, perhaps, elsewhere.

Choriocarcinoma is exceptionally aggressive. It grows explosively, invading and destroying surrounding tissue, and it metastasizes readily, to the brain, lung, liver, and elsewhere. It's also astonishingly responsive to radiation and chemotherapy: More than half of all patients with metastatic choriocarcinoma are cured. Yanira's doctors began treatment immediately. Within weeks her beta hCG blood levels were negligible, a sign that no trace of the tumor remained.

In the four years since, Yanira experienced no recurrence. Her doctors consider her cured. But her brain damage was catastrophic and permanent. Months spent in rehab facilities have made no difference. She wears diapers and can't see, walk, or wash. She's mentally competent in the eyes of the law, but only minimally so. "She says she's going to finish school," Iris told me. "She wants to go to college to learn a trade. That's her thinking—the doctors say she's not going to get much better. There's nothing they can really do for her. They've told her that."

And Yanira has lost custody of her daughter. She signed papers to this effect, according to Iris, several months after she finished her cancer treatment. Her former fiancé's sister now has legal custody, and the two of them share child care duties uneasily with Iris. Iris is convinced that her granddaughter's dad, who she says did time for dealing crack, is selling on the streets again and is a bad influence. Yanira wants custody back but isn't up to its burdens. "My daughter knows that she has a daughter," Iris told me, "and she wants to see her all the time. But she cannot take care of her."

Had Yanira's cancer been caught before it spread to her brain, she'd almost surely have averted any lasting effects. And had it been detected just a few days earlier, before her fall and the downward movement of her brain, she might, at worst, have suffered some sensory loss or muscle weakness. Radiation and chemotherapy would have destroyed the cancer in her brain, perhaps abetted by surgery to remove some of the tumor's bulk. The catastrophic event was her brain's downward shift, or herniation, into her spinal column. This destroyed large areas of living tissue, through a combination of trauma, as her brain pressed against bone, and cut-off of oxygen, as large arteries were squeezed shut. Intervention to shrink her tumor's mass and relieve the pressure in her skull during the days or hours before the downward shift would have prevented it.

Had the ER doctors at Episcopal or Northeastern ordered a head CT or MRI to assess Yanira's headaches, numbness, and right-side weakness, they'd have discovered the dire situation in time to act. Had Dr. Davies at Northeastern ordered follow-up imaging to resolve the mystery of the "pregnancy without a fetus" found on ultrasound, he'd have discovered the undiagnosed choriocarcinoma in her uterus—and probably figured that the ferocity of this tumor type meant a high likelihood of spread to other organs. And had he suspected metastatic cancer, he'd almost certainly have seen her weakness and numbness in a more suspicious light. They're classic symptoms of localized brain injury—harm of the sort doctors expect from a tumor. Yanira's nausea, vomiting, and headaches fit the picture as well. They're the standard signs of elevated intracranial pressure—pressure that forced her brain's downward shift. Follow-on studies of Yanira's womb would thus have nudged the diagnostic workup in a different direction, toward brain scans that could have caught her tumor in time to avert disaster.

Doctors don't think systematically; they recognize patterns on the fly, amid competing demands on their attention. And they react to these patterns—by ordering tests and prescribing treatments—in ways shaped by resource constraints that they take for granted. In the barely controlled chaos of a big-city ER, they act on reflex, without time to ponder the underlying premises. But these premises drive decisions, and they reflect limitations on the availability of equipment (and people to run it) in hospitals burdened by large numbers of patients who cannot pay. They also reflect the busyness and the distractions—the manic intensity—of the urban ER, and the consequent impossibility of in-depth consideration of each patient's case.

Physicians adjust their practice styles, often unconsciously, to fit these constraints on clinical resources and to manage the myriad demands on their attention. In so doing, they strike tacit balances between benefit and cost, tolerating risk to life and health. They thus impose limits on society's behalf, a role at odds with the Hippocratic ideal of undivided loyalty to patients. But they're loath to admit this, even to themselves.

The Tacit Balancing of Benefits and Costs

In the malpractice suit that followed Yanira's life-changing misfortune, her lawyer portrayed the Episcopal and Northeastern ER doctors as both aware and uncaring about the danger she faced. But the doctors' responses to questions at trial reveal a more confused understanding. On cross-examination, Yanira's doctor at Episcopal, Sean Lenahan, conceded that her story of headaches, numbness, and right-side weakness raised the possibility of a brain tumor, a possibility he could have explored with a more thorough (and time-consuming) physical exam. And he admitted that a head CT scan would have found the tumor he missed—in time to save her.

Yet Dr. Lenahan insisted he'd ruled a brain tumor out. His physical exam was a good-enough basis for doing so, he claimed, since he didn't find the numbness or weakness she'd described. He didn't order a CT scan, he explained, because he "didn't feel that there was any abnormalit[y] that warranted" one.

Dr. Lenahan could have argued that the vast majority of young women who come to the ER complaining of nausea, vomiting, and headache are suffering from minor ailments not meriting a CT scan's expense. And he might have tried to justify giving Yanira's complaints of weakness and numbness less weight because he couldn't confirm them on physical exam. Consider some simple numbers. Suppose the CT scan costs $500, and Yanira's doctors think she has a one in a hundred chance of having a readily treatable tumor, detectable on CT. That's $50,000 per tumor diagnosed ($500 for the CT scan times 100 scans)—pricey but surely worth it, to avert catastrophic brain damage. But now add some zeros, say two, to her probability of having the tumor. This ups the cost per tumor found to $5 million ($500 for the CT times 10,000 scans), roughly the "value of life"—$5 million to $10 million—calculated by economists from consumers' and workers' decisions about how much money they'll pay or forgo to avoid deadly risk.[29] Add another zero, and the cost per tumor found rises to $50 million—not worth it, according to these economists' studies, and a deadly misuse of resources since more people could be saved by spending this money on other things.

So Dr. Lenahan could have argued that a head CT wasn't worth doing, not because a brain tumor had been "ruled out," but because its cost outweighed its low likelihood of finding something important. But this would have required him to admit—to Yanira's lawyer, the jury, and himself—that he weighed society's (or the hospital's) interests against his patient's, something not permitted by the Hippocratic Oath. This he could not, or would not, do. Instead, he clung to two contradictory propositions: that he'd "ruled out" a brain tumor on physical exam and that a CT would have found the tumor and saved Yanira.

Yanira's other ER doctors were similarly avoidant about the balance between cost and risk that they'd tacitly struck. Her lawyer, Ken Rothweiler, worked this with devastating effect. Dr. Davies, who saw her during her second visit to Northeastern, didn't claim to have "ruled out" a tumor. But on cross-examination, he insisted that his clinical history and physical were "correct" and "would not allow me to predict that she had a brain tumor":

> At no time did I think she had a brain tumor. I had a first trimester pregnant woman with nausea and vomiting, normal neurological examination, no headache. And another reason [pregnancy], a very good reason for the nausea and vomiting. It would have been—it would have been wrong of me to order a CAT scan at that time. No reasonable physician in an emergency room setting would have ordered a CAT scan on the patient that I saw that night.

Rothweiler seized the moment:

> Oh, really? Well, the next day when she came into Temple they ordered a CAT scan after she fell down the 13 steps. Are you saying that that physician wasn't reasonable?

Rothweiler was being cagey here, of course: the patient brought to Temple, unresponsive, after she'd tumbled down a flight of stairs wasn't the same person Davies had seen hours earlier. What had changed were the probabilities. At Temple, after the fall, the chance was high that something awful was going on inside Yanira's head. At Northeastern, Yanira was awake and alert, with other explanations, much more likely than a brain tumor, for her headache, nausea, and vomiting. Dr. Davies reasonably treated the likelihood of a brain tumor as low and tacitly judged the potential yield from a CT as insufficient to merit the expense. But had he said so to the jury—had he admitted to putting cost concerns ahead of his patient's life chances—he'd have done violence to jurors' Hippocratic expectations. By characterizing his failure to order the CT as a right-or-wrong question rather than a judgment about clinical costs and probabilities, he could avert doing so.

But by going this route, he barred himself from arguing that he'd made a sensible decision about the balance of cost and probability. He was thus a setup for Rothweiler's attack: If probabilities are beside the point, how could a CT scan have been necessary when Yanira was brought to Temple but "wrong" at Northeastern, hours before?

Negligence law, of which medical malpractice law is a subspecies, embraces the balancing of probabilities. It requires actors to take precautions when the benefits of doing so outweigh the burdens, and it holds them liable when they don't.[30] Over the past few decades, courts have increasingly defined this duty in economics language. They've said all of us have an obligation to take steps less costly than the harms we'd prevent, discounted by the probability of these harms occurring. But medical malpractice is an awkward exception. The law embraces the Hippocratic premise that doctors don't compromise their patients' interests to conserve society's resources. Judges don't ask jurors to weigh clinical costs and benefits; they instruct jurors to defer to doctors' opinions about the appropriate standard of care. Juries have discretion to choose between competing medical experts' opinions, but they must accept a doctor's testimony when it's not contradicted by another's.

The law thus embraces, indeed reinforces, medicine's unwillingness to overtly compromise patients' life chances so as to conserve resources. Such compromise, though, is cloaked within clinical practice norms. The practice protocols that Dr. Lenahan cited in his defense—protocols adopted by the American College of Emergency Physicians—require particular findings on physical exam to trigger the ordering of a CT scan: These include neck stiffness (a sign of meningitis), localized weakness or loss of sensation, and sudden changes in personality or cognitive ability.[31] Headache alone is not enough, and a patient's account of her symptoms, unverified by a doctor's exam, is deemed iffy as a basis for scheduling a CT. On the witness stand, Dr. Davies cited radiation exposure as a reason for his reluctance. But the lifetime risk of cancer from a single head CT prescribed for a twenty-year-old is trivial—about 1 in 10,000.[32] Embedded in the practice protocols Dr. Lenahan drew upon is concern about soaring medical costs and willingness to play the percentages accordingly.

Lenahan was reluctant to admit this to a jury, or to himself. Doctors, though, sometimes fess up to counting costs. In a teaching manual, a professor of emergency medicine at the Medical College of Georgia urges students to "recognize the problem":

> Cost containment will eventually effect us all. The way we practice medicine in the future depends on what we collectively do today. We must learn what the minimum appropriate work-up is for every illness and discipline ourselves to order only those tests or interventions absolutely necessary. If we are used to ordering a CT scan for every patient in the ED [Emergency Department] with a headache, eventually, there will be no place for us in the modern health care system![33]

But the professor, Walter Kuhn, also put his students on notice about the competing pressures that operate covertly: "I, myself, have often said, 'They pay me to be right, not cheap.' In the long run we need to be right *and* cheap."[34]

Unspoken trade-offs between being "right" and being "cheap" are embedded in myriad protocols followed by doctors in all specialties. You've almost surely been treated, evaluated, or screened for disease in accordance with guidelines that put you at avoidable risk in order to reduce costs. Protocols concerning colonoscopy to screen for bowel cancers, mammography and MRI to search for breast tumors, and use of "statin" drugs to slow atherosclerosis are everyday examples. The doctors who draft these protocols are open about the *health* risks these tests and treatments impose, but they speak in euphemism, if at all, about the weight they give to costs.

The debate over use of MRI to detect early breast cancer is illustrative. There's mounting evidence that MRI finds tiny malignancies more effectively than mammography, albeit with frequent false-positives (results that require follow-up studies to rule out cancer). But mammograms run from $50 to $150, while breast MRIs cost fifteen times more. Among medical opinion leaders, there's much discussion of the false-positive problem (even though mammograms produce plenty of false positives) but only coded reference to relative price as a reason to limit the role of MRI.

A recent *New England Journal of Medicine* editorial on the subject, by the American Cancer Society's chief developer of screening guidelines, barely hints at the gap in price yet gives it decisive weight. "The responsible use of MRI for the evaluation of the breast is focused primarily on patients with a high probability of breast cancer,"[35] the author opines. The Cancer Society's "Guidelines for Breast Screening with MRI as an Adjunct to Mammography" go a bit further, citing costs per quality-adjusted life year for women in high-risk groups.[36] For these women—patients with worrisome family histories, dangerous genes, or previous breast tumors—the cost per quality-adjusted life year is clearly worth paying, assuming, as economists do, that the "value of life" is $5 to $10 million. The "Guidelines" set a rough risk threshold: They support annual MRI screening for women with a 20 to 25 percent or greater lifetime risk of developing breast cancer. But what about women with, say, an average lifetime risk of breast cancer—about 15 percent? The "Guidelines" do *not* recommend MRI screening for them. The authors don't speak to the question of whether the higher cost per life year for these women is worth paying. But they answer this question with a tacit "no." This frees insurers to say "no" to coverage of

MRI screening for women who aren't in high-risk groups,[37] and it signals their doctors not to prescribe it.[38]

Quiet and Gentle Hypocrisy?

Veiled sacrifice of patients' survival prospects in order to save money is increasingly a feature of clinical practice near the end of life. Gone are the days when most disputes over the continuation of life-sustaining treatment pitted family members eager to stop the full-court press against doctors intent on continuing it. Today, the roles more typically are reversed: Physicians resist providing care they deem futile, while family members want everything done. Several years ago, I was asked to speak on end-of-life issues at an ethics retreat for physicians at a large, West Coast HMO. One case seized my attention—the story of Sara Eisenberg,[39] an 82-year-old woman who suffered a massive heart attack while visiting her daughter. She arrived at the hospital short of breath, with crushing chest pain, and her blood pressure quickly dropped to dangerous levels. Tests showed that blockages in her coronary arteries had destroyed the front wall of her left ventricle, the heart's main pumping chamber. Mrs. Eisenberg was admitted to intensive care, then put on pressors—intravenous medications that boost blood pressure by causing muscle cells surrounding tiny arteries to contract, just as shutting off faucets and fire hydrants raises water pressure. Her cardiologist quickly concluded that her prognosis was dismal, a view the intensive care team shared. Aggressive doses of pressors failed to raise her systolic pressure above 70 (a worrisome prognostic sign), while putting her at risk for destruction of organs dependent on adequate blood flow. Yet she remained awake, alert, and chatty. "She was the littlest, tiniest Jewish grandmother you ever saw," a hospital social worker recalled. And when her doctors told her she wasn't going to make it, she nodded her head but didn't believe it.

Sara's daughter Lisa,[40] a lawyer, was around when the doctors delivered this dire prognosis. "Her daughter felt it was an assault," the social worker told me. "She couldn't understand why they [the doctors] each felt compelled to repeat these comments—to tell her mother she should be making plans." Lisa began paying close attention to clinical details. She tracked treatment plans, followed lab values, and questioned the doctors about their intentions. "She knew what the doses of each of the pressors was, what the blood pressure was." Each time the treatment team tried to withdraw pressors, Lisa's suspicions rose. The doctors, in turn, grew annoyed. Some resorted to the language of psychopathology. "It felt to me like there was a fairly strong codependency between mother and daughter," Sara's cardiologist recalled. "Her daughter could not let go, even in the face of a bad prognosis. She was taking . . . an adversarial position, almost litigious. . . . What I tried to clarify for her was that this was not an adversarial relationship."

But in his conversations with me, Sara's cardiologist admitted to some thinking that wouldn't have reassured Lisa: "When we see dollars wasted, that's not a good thing. Nobody presents that to the patient. . . . The problem is that individual members only care about themselves, because they don't have the global perspective." The HMO's doctors, he told me, reinforce each other's sense of this broader perspective: "There's an acculturation within the organization that happens at different speeds for different people. There's a very strong group identity and a very strong sense of being guardians of the resources and needing to use them wisely in order to preserve them for the greater good." "Without any question," he said, "we are subconsciously rationing care, whether we call it that or believe that's what we're doing. . . . If we didn't, the reality is that we would be facing an absurdity in which we made . . . near-futile efforts to save one life out of an enormous number of failures. We'd bankrupt our health care system." But, he acknowledged, he and his colleagues had no answer to the question of how to square this with Hippocratic ideals.

It's hardly surprising that doctors often seek an easier way out. The care at issue, they're wont to say, is futile. It inflicts misery in pursuit of wishful thinking. After Sara's first few days in the hospital, this became the prevailing view among her caregivers. "We agreed that her prognosis was quite dismal for functional survival," her cardiologist recalled. Her cardiac ejection fraction, a measure of the heart's ability to pump blood, hovered on the margins of viability. Each time the ICU team tried to taper her pressors, her blood pressure dropped to levels incompatible with life. Meanwhile, continued high doses of these powerful medications were putting her vital organs at growing risk. And there were the many small agonies of ICU treatment— the tube in Sara's bladder, the bright lights and beeping monitors, and the catheter threaded through an incision in her neck, into a vein and toward her heart. "My staff was very upset," the cardiologist recounted. "It was their impression that the patient was suffering on an ongoing basis and that the daughter did not want to let go—and that the patient was going along to please her daughter."

Once, while Sara's cardiologist was away from the hospital, a covering doctor spoke too candidly. Colleagues reported that he came into Sara's ICU cubicle, told her she didn't have enough working heart muscle to survive, and then asked, "Have you ever stayed in a really expensive hotel, like the Plaza?" Sara replied with something like, "Yeah, guess so." The doctor then ventured, "Well, you know how expensive a room is? Six to eight hundred dollars. Well, you know how expensive *this* room is? Ten thousand dollars." Lisa was in the room all the while. She became furious. She threatened to sue, demanded new doctors, and insisted that all be done to keep her mom alive. Sara's terrified caregivers agreed to go all-out, though some complained quietly and bitterly about the waste of resources.

Four weeks later, Sara left the hospital on foot. She was successfully weaned from pressors without damage to her kidneys or other organs, then transferred from the ICU to a regular floor to prepare her for discharge. Her ejection fraction—in the low 20s on admission, barely enough to support life—soared to 35 percent, an inexplicable development since cardiac muscle that dies during a heart attack doesn't regenerate. Her doctors had no scientific explanation for her recovery.[41] "I was flabbergasted," Sara's cardiologist told me. "I've been doing this for close to twenty years now—you try to develop a sense of whether a patient who is quite ill has a chance of surviving. . . . For me, the bottom line is that this case speaks so much to our inability to prognosticate and how helpless we are to guide people in any reliable way."

After her discharge, Sara divided her time between her daughter's home, an assisted living facility, and her own residence. There were some rocky medical moments, including a rehospitalization for fluid in her lungs after aides gave her the wrong diet and her kidneys failed to clear excess water and salt. But Lisa enjoyed the gift of years with her mom that she'd figured, for a terrifying week, weren't to be. Her kids gained all the intangibles of having, as a grandmom, a tiny, sweet, spunky old lady who never gives up. And Sara had the joy that comes with giving these gifts—and knowing that she beat the odds.

"It's that kind of experience that makes it very difficult for me to ever tell a patient, 'You have a zero chance of survival,'" her cardiologist reflected. But his failure to get the prognosis right wasn't his main regret. Alluding to his colleague's remarks comparing Sara's ICU stay to time spent at the Plaza Hotel, he offered:

> Had the comments not been made, . . . I would be willing to wager that in a few days, I would have been able to convince the family that enough was enough, and she would have ended up dying fairly rapidly . . . and none of this would have come to the forefront.

The remarks were, he said, "asinine—you never say that type of thing to a family." But stopping the pressors and letting Sara die would have been the right thing to do, since the chance of success was so small compared to the cost:

> The reality is that this happens every day. . . . An enormous number of people go through their lives and go to the hospital and die every day, because you don't have something that comes up that disrupts the doctor-patient relationship. . . . If you say that for every eighty or ninety year old lady—if you say that the fact that this lady survived means we should do that type of thing for every patient—I'm not prepared to say that.

So his main regret about Sara's case, he told me, was the breakdown in relations between Sara (and Lisa) and her doctors. "The patient-physician relationship is a really critical thing, and here a disruption of that relationship was a really critical thing in our ability to take care of this patient." About rationing at the bedside, he said, "We should continue to be quietly and gently hypocritical."

Opportunities to be "quietly and gently hypocritical" are expanding. Most states let doctors refuse to provide treatment that's "futile" or not "appropriate." The ambiguous meaning of these terms has discouraged doctors and hospitals from taking full advantage—they're afraid of getting sued[42]— but the trend line has been toward greater willingness to say no. Professional and academic commentators—in medicine, bioethics, and law—increasingly speak of "medical futility" as a reason not to treat.[43] A 1999 Texas statute, much-praised as a model, empowers hospitals to stop treatment that's "futile" without fear of liability, so long as ethics consultants sign off on the treatment team's determination of "futility."[44] The Texas law doesn't define "futility," leaving this up to the ethics consultants, who are often hospital employees; nor have the boundaries of "futility" been clearly drawn by professional bodies or the courts. This silence has created a sheltered legal space for saying no to pricey care that's potentially life-saving.

The "poster children" for the medical futility movement have been clearly hopeless situations—cases like Terry Schiavo's a decade ago. Schiavo was famously kept alive for years in a persistent vegetative state without hope of regaining consciousness. The notion of "futility," though, has been expanding to encompass cases like Sara's—situations in which a positive outcome *seems* improbable but can't be ruled out. Some physicians now embrace a proposition advanced by ethicist Lawrence Schneiderman—that therapies with a less than 1 percent chance of success[45] should be deemed futile.[46] But the 1 percent solution is more metaphor than decision rule since the complexity and uniqueness of each case precludes exactness about outcomes.

A few commentators openly endorse the covert withholding of life-saving care. Doctors, argues ethicist and legal scholar Mark Hall, should tap their patients' trust as a "resource," to be employed on behalf of the common good.[47] Hall lays out a line of reasoning that makes some stomachs queasy— and that closely tracks what Sara's cardiologist had to say. The gist is that patients' trust in their doctors is "resilient": people who are sick and afraid tend to become childlike in their need for a champion who'll stand by them. So when clinical circumstances turn dire, their skepticism wanes and their trust deepens—whether or not caregivers are trust*worthy*. Doctors, Hall says, should seize this opportunity to set limits furtively. Their sickest patients' neediness empowers them to do so without inviting suspicion.

Hall, in other words, countenances doctors' betrayal of their Hippocratic commitment on the ground that they're unlikely to be found out. It's an intrepid line of argument, rather like saying a spouse's affair isn't a problem so long as her life partner is trusting enough to miss any hints of it. But it captures an emerging sense among doctors caught between Hippocratic expectations and pressure to limit use of costly tests and treatments. Acknowledging the role of cost in life-and-death decisions isn't a viable option, Sara's cardiologist told me. "The very idea that we'd do that in this marketplace—we lost 2,000 members last month"—is, he insisted, absurd. "To further alarm people with, 'you can't always get what you want'—it's not exactly a marketing strategy."

But being "quietly and gently hypocritical" has its risks. For one, hypocrisy of this sort breeds self-deception as doctors cling to the belief that they're honoring Hippocratic ideals. Sara's doctors convinced themselves that she wanted life-sustaining efforts to stop (despite her insistence to the contrary), that her daughter was putting unconscionable pressure on her to go along with these efforts, and that everyone was on the same side—they weren't in an "adversarial relationship" with Sara and Lisa. At the same time, they professed (to me) a commitment to stewardship of limited resources with an eye toward the greater good, even if it meant sacrificing Sara's chances for life. This brew of contradictions boiled over when one of her doctors broached the question of cost by casting her ICU stay as akin to a night at The Plaza.

Doctors do the work of being "quietly and gently hypocritical" by bending their understandings of reality—both their patients' realities and their own—to reduce the anxiety that accompanies cognitive dissonance. But the anxiety seeps out, sometimes as sarcasm or anger, signaling to patients and their families that something is amiss. And the bent perceptions—beliefs that *patients* want to stop costly therapies or that a treatment's prospects for success are zero, rather than modest and uncertain—are occasionally exposed by events as false. That's what happened in Sara's case, shattering relations between her daughter and her doctors. We're hard-wired to believe that hypocrisy is wrong—and to be wounded and angered by unfaithfulness when we're on the receiving end.[48]

Silence about the counting of costs also precludes reasoned deliberation about how to do so. It stifles conversation about how to weigh health care's incommensurable benefits—life's quality as well as its length, patients' grasp of why bad things have happened and what might lie ahead, and the feeling of not being alone in the path of fate. Practice protocols (like those for use of MRI to detect breast cancer) that rest on undiscussed valuations of life risk treating sufferers of different diseases inconsistently and thus unfairly. And case-by-case clinical judgments tied to physicians' prejudices about the worth of particular lives are a recipe for injustice. Failure to formulate overt cost-benefit trade-off policies also frees health care stakeholders—drug and device makers, medical specialty societies, and patients with particular diseases—to contend for resources without needing to take account of the wider social perspective. The path of "quiet and gentle hypocrisy," in short, is a route through a landscape of unreason, inequity, and covert bias.

About the biases at play—the masked moral and political content of medical practice norms—I'll have more to say in chapter 4. I turn now to the question of what Washington's health policy makers can do to control costs without calling upon our doctors to break faith.

chapter three

stakeholders, wonks, and the setting of limits

Washington's Wishful Thinking: Controlling Costs by Cutting Waste

It would be wonderful if we could contain medical costs by selectively eliminating care that yields no clinical benefits. That's what Washington's health reformers keep promising. Withholding care that saves lives in order to save money is as unspeakable in Congress as it is at the bedside. And yes, there's some truth to what I was asked to say as an Obama surrogate about opportunities to slash medical spending that buys us nothing. There's the 30 percent of health spending that's wasted on worthless care[1]—about the price of the $700 billion mortgage bailout, squandered each year. Plus there's the 10 percent or so of medical spending that covers avoidable administrative costs—another $200 billion a year. It surely makes sense to target this spending, by learning more about which tests and treatments work, cutting out those that don't, and getting rid of pointless bureaucracy.

But cutting out the care that's useless is astonishingly difficult. Most people think that doctors know which tests and treatments do and don't work—for most patients, at least. So did I, until it dawned on me a few months into medical school that my pediatrician had put one over on me by telling me he knew his nostrums would help. I'd fled, as an eight-year-old, from his allergy shots—under the examining table, up some stairs, and into a closet out of his reach. And, it turns out, the sorcerer's mix of mold, pollen, and mammal hairs he injected into me weekly, when he could catch me, hasn't been shown to work, notwithstanding the hundreds of dollars my parents spent on the stuff. My medical professors challenged me and my fellow first-years to insist on proof—and showed us that many of the treatments in common use do nothing. The same year, the Office of Technology Assessment (an agency that advised Congress on scientific questions until it was shut down in 1995) estimated that only about 10 to 20 percent of medical procedures rest on "gold-standard" evidence—randomized clinical trials.[2]

It's doubtful that this percentage has changed much in the thirty years since. The challenges are daunting. Drug companies, makers of medical devices, and clinical specialty societies fiercely resist efforts to compare tests and treatments and to condition payment on proof of effectiveness. There are classic horror stories, including that of the back surgeons who arched their backs when a federal agency empowered to make science-based treatment recommendations concluded that evidence favored fewer spinal operations for lower-back pain.[3] Facing down this threat, they convinced Congress to geld the agency by barring it from issuing clinical guidance.[4]

A more recent example is so-called "CT angiography," which sums up serial, CT slices of the heart to create stunning three-dimensional views of clogged (or clear) coronary arteries. These images allow a glimpse inside the heart without so much as a needle stick. But whether this look enables doctors to save lives is uncertain. Their use soared in 2006, after General Electric brought high-resolution, 64-slice scanners to market. Medicare officials became alarmed about the cost.[5] In December 2007, the agency that runs Medicare said it would pay for the scans only in limited circumstances and only if the doctors who did them participated in studies of their effectiveness.[6] Physicians who'd invested in the machines went to war, demanding that Medicare cover the scans without condition. They lobbied Congress (as did GE), getting 79 Members to sign onto a letter asking the agency to pay for them without limitation.[7] Three months after its December announcement, Medicare reversed course, saying it would cover the test without restrictions and offering only "hope" for future studies of the scans' effectiveness.

Risky and pricey therapies routinely make their way into common use without such studies.[8] Recent examples include hormone replacement for post-menopausal women and use of tiny screens coated with anti-clotting drugs to prop open coronary arteries; both treatments made headlines when federally funded clinical trials found that they killed more people than they saved.[9] Another federally funded study, also conducted after-the-fact, revealed that a whole family of new, patent-protected antipsychotic drugs, adopted by most psychiatrists in the 1990s in response to aggressive marketing, performed no better than cheap, generic medications.[10]

What was most remarkable about these episodes was that rigorous studies were eventually done. The CT angiography story is more typical: new technologies stream into the market with minimal attention to their comparative efficacy. Private insurers won't pay for such studies for reasons that are right out of Economics 101: a finding that a therapy is ineffective benefits *all* insurers, not just the firm that funded it. Comparative effectiveness research is, in economics lingo, a "public good"—its results are available to all (through publication) and so can't be used by one health plan to get a leg up on its rivals.

Change is looming. The 2010 health reform law created a "Patient-Centered Outcomes Research Institute," funded by levies on Medicare and private insurers, to sponsor such research. But the funding level, less than a tenth of a percent of what Americans spend on health care each year, will do little to increase the fraction of medical decisions that rest on science. And the Institute's governing body—composed mostly of representatives from the hospital, insurance, and drug and device industries, as well as physicians—seems almost designed to enable stakeholders to block studies that threaten their interests. Moreover, multiple provisions in the law (sought by providers and drug and device makers) hobble Medicare's ability to base coverage decisions on research the Institute sponsors.[11]

Even when researchers show that a treatment is both better and cheaper, stakeholders who stand to lose if doctors follow the data often use their clout to ensure that doctors don't. A case in point is the "Allhat" study,[12] a landmark clinical trial of drugs oft-prescribed to reduce heart attack and stroke risk for tens of millions of Americans with high blood pressure. In this study, a fifty-year-old diuretic (a pill that coaxes the kidneys to make more urine)—available for fifty cents a week—outperformed several patent-protected drugs costing many times more.[13] One of these drugs, Pfizer's "Cardura," a chemical that relaxes blood vessels by blocking the action of so-called "alpha" receptors, nearly doubled its recipients' risk of heart failure, compared to the diuretic, prompting the "Allhat" researchers to drop it from the trial in 2000, two years before they published their results. Another Pfizer product, its best-selling calcium channel blocker "Norvasc," increased heart failure risk by nearly 40 percent, at a price twenty times higher than the diuretic.

Pfizer responded by instructing its sales force on strategies to reassure doctors that "Cardura" was safe and by spinning "Allhat" as a "Norvasc" success story, a feat accomplished by noting that "Norvasc" and the diuretic achieved similar reductions in *heart attack* and *stroke* risk—and by ignoring the heart failure numbers.[14] One executive boasted in an e-mail that Pfizer reps kept key clinical opinion leaders away from a conference presentation on "Allhat" by "sending [them] to sightsee."[15]

Pfizer went further, paying $200,000 in 2003 to one of the study's leaders, Dr. Richard Grimm. Grimm gave a series of talks to doctors suggesting that diuretics were no better than their pricier rivals, including "Norvasc," and he led a campaign to oust a "Norvasc" skeptic as chair of the study's steering committee.[16] In all, Pfizer spent millions to promote "Norvasc," winning over key opinion leaders, making doctors familiar with it through advertising and detailing, and overwhelming the federal Heart, Lung, & Blood Institute's efforts to advocate diuretics. The unsurprising result was that "Norvasc" sales surged, to nearly $5 billion in 2006. Sales dipped the next year, when "Norvasc" lost patent protection and Pfizer dialed down its promotional efforts.[17] But diuretics didn't take up the slack. Instead, newer, patent-protected medicines, not on the market when "Allhat" was designed, filled the void, without being put to the test of comparative efficacy.

The "Allhat" affair illustrates the limits of researcher's ability to influence clinical practice. Not only are powerful stakeholders able to resist the findings; research can't keep pace with the appearance of new therapies and the eclipse of others for business reasons. The expiration of Pfizer's "Norvasc" patent, not the drug's poor clinical trial performance, explains its 2007 decline in use. Another "Allhat" loser, AstraZeneca's "Zestril,"[18] also went off-patent, reducing AstraZeneca's interest in promoting it. Meanwhile, a new drug, "Diovan," part of a chemical family not studied in "Allhat," emerged as a leader in the high-stakes contest for America's hypertensives. In 2007, "Diovan" sales reached $5 billion, eclipsing the economic performance of all the "Allhat" competitors. The marketplace had left "Allhat" behind.

Even when research data stamp a test or treatment as a clear loser, its proponents can point to variation among patients as reason for continuing to pitch it. There's a fractal geometry of clinical differences—an endless variation in patients' responses to pathogens, pills, and procedures. So it's just about always possible to argue, "Our patients are different"—different enough to benefit from a therapy that's been proven inferior for the population as a whole. Doctors, drugmakers, and others are already seizing upon the promise of "personalized medicine"—the science-based tailoring of care to individual patients. It's a promise worth pursuing. But we're nowhere near to a grasp of the protean interactions between genetic and environmental influences that shape our susceptibilities to disease and treatment. Biological understanding of this sort is probably centuries away—remote because of our ignorance about how genes and environmental stimuli sculpt our anatomy and physiology. Indeed, such an understanding could forever elude us: complex, interactive systems like weather, economies, and the physiology of higher life forms may be inherently unpredictable.[19]

So the 30 percent of health spending that's squandered on useless services is an implausible source of large, near-term savings. The same is the case for the 10 percent or more of medical spending that's wasted on excess administration. We're not about to shift to a Canadian-style "single-payer" system, able to slash administrative costs to half or a third of current levels. Stakeholder resistance[20] and popular antipathy to centralized power will ensure the survival of our fragmented approach to health care financing. This fragmented system, featuring multiple insurers and myriad coverage approaches, means more administrative complexity.

Even if it were possible to slash the *entirety* of the 30 percent spent on useless care, *plus* the 10 percent spent on excess administration, the resulting savings would pale by comparison with the cost control challenge ahead. Suppose (implausibly!) that a package of reforms could eliminate *all* of this waste—now, 40 percent of health spending—within five years. This would cut medical spending by 8 percentage points, on average, during each of the five years. That's a formidable accomplishment, but it would only temporarily offset the 5 to 10 percent annual increase in health spending that's been a near-constant over the past few decades. We'd delay the reckoning for several years, but we wouldn't avert it—unless we take steps to nudge the curve of rising costs downward over the long haul.

Getting to "No," Gently

How might we "bend the curve"[21] without pushing doctors to break faith—with their patients and with Hippocratic ideals? We need to start by acknowledging both that bending the curve will require the foregoing of care that saves lives and that "quiet hypocrisy" about this isn't a viable option. Our nation's long-term fiscal stability will turn on whether we can find a way to say no without provoking popular anger that makes naysaying impossible. We've thus far failed miserably at this challenge. But there is a way forward—one that leverages human psychology, market pressures, and the law to achieve much greater frugality without breaking faith at the bedside.

Let's begin with some psychology—specifically, the psychology of rescue. We're hard-wired to respond to people in dire straits by doing our utmost to help them.[22] In the film *Saving Private Ryan,* the larger ends of war dissolve as a platoon takes senseless risks to find a lost soldier—senseless, that is, if one disregards the combat deaths of his three brothers just days before. That this family catastrophe is special—special enough to provoke General George Marshall to order his commanders to find Ryan and "get him the hell out of there"—is the film's central trope. Men die as the quest unfolds. That the war is against the Nazis seems beside the point; the soldiers' sacrifice is ennobled by their devotion to each other.

We revere those who undertake rescue at great cost. We judge people harshly when they have the chance to do so and they don't. Medicine's Hippocratic commitment is of a piece with this sentiment. But we're not inclined toward similar blame when the lives at stake are statistical abstractions or when circumstances appear to make rescue impossible. We don't, for example, judge our doctors harshly when they fail to deliver the cures "Dr. McCoy" provides on *Star Trek*. We don't scorn the cardiologists of the 1980s for their inattention to blood lipid levels now known to cause coronary vascular disease. And we're not angry at today's heart specialists for their failure to provide therapies, yet to be discovered, that might someday dissolve killer arterial plaque just as antibiotics today cure deadly infections.

This suggests a strategy for slowing the growth of health spending without counting on our doctors to betray us covertly. We ought to make it much harder for new, high-cost tests and treatments to become part of our expectations as patients. We can't (and shouldn't) stop scientific progress: the quest to better understand our biological selves is both part of who we are and a font for future improvements in human well-being. But we can and should distinguish between decisive advances—scientific breakthroughs that make large therapeutic leaps possible—and what the physician and philosopher of science Lewis Thomas called "halfway technologies"[23]—interventions that are, at once, sophisticated from an engineering perspective and crude in their action upon human physiology.

Interventions of the latter sort are the main culprits behind soaring costs. They employ pricey personnel to run sophisticated equipment. And because this equipment is a substitute, not a fix, for physiology gone wrong, it's often employed for extended periods. The beeping machines in intensive care units are characteristic. Respirators, intra-cardiac monitors, portable scanners, and other state-of-the-art technologies run up the bill during our last weeks and months while typically doing little to put our biology back on track. Our system of paying for health care bestows rich rewards on those who develop these technologies and learn to use them, whether the therapeutic gains are large or trivial.

By contrast, breakthroughs in *biological* understanding lead to larger clinical advances that cost less. The antibiotic revolution is a classic example. The discovery that substances found in nature (and later synthesized in the lab) could stop bacterial growth by blocking key chemical reactions was a finding of extraordinary elegance. A more recent instance is the elucidation of the pathways of lipid metabolism in the 1970s by two Texas scientists, Joseph Goldstein and Michael Brown. This understanding opened the way for chemical intervention to slow the synthesis of artery-clogging combinations of lipids and proteins. The "statin" drugs, which reduce levels of dangerous, low-density lipoprotein and thereby slow the growth of arterial plaque, are an early fruit of this understanding. Antibiotics and statins are remarkably cheap by comparison with the technologies employed in intensive care units. They interact in sophisticated ways with biological systems to set them right. The science that spawns such advances is worth supporting. But the technologies that *substitute* for physiology gone wrong, rather than setting it right, merit more tepid backing. They play minor roles in health improvement, and they're mainly responsible for medicine's rising costs.

So we should make it much harder than it is now for new, "halfway" technologies to reach the market. That way, doctors won't break faith with their patients by failing to provide them. We can start by pushing for proof of superior therapeutic value before covering new treatments and thereby incorporating them into clinical practice. The stakeholders that stand to lose—medical device-makers, specialists, and others for whom halfway measures yield fulsome profits—have resisted such requirements with great success. But as costs rise—and as businesses, taxpayers, and America's creditors become less tolerant—these stakeholders' leverage will decline.

More important are the reward systems that today favor technological wizardry over biological breakthroughs—or time spent speaking with patients or thinking through their problems. I recall doing some simple math, while a medical student on a surgery rotation, and figuring out that my attending made more money per minute for time spent in the operating room than the actress Debra Winger made doing her steamy scenes in that year's hit film, *An Officer and a Gentleman.* He took in $7,000 a case from Medicare for coronary bypass surgery, and on some mornings he'd have two cases going at once, in adjacent operating rooms. He could pull this off because his eager residents and fellows, counting on the same payoffs someday, did almost all of each case, from "cracking" the chest (to open it) to closing up ribs and muscle when work on the heart was done. My attending would put in only about 20 minutes on each case, sewing in some of the little leg veins used to bypass blocked arteries. Had he spent this time talking with patients, he'd have taken home perhaps a few hundred dollars.

This financial preference for invasive, halfway measures pervades American medicine. Practitioners who perform them take home much more than doctors who dispense statins, antibiotics, and other technologically simpler therapies, even when these therapies are more biologically sophisticated and effective.[24] Hospitals likewise earn much more from insurers for invasive, high-tech services. This, in turn, makes doctors and hospitals more willing to pay for pricey equipment and for employees to run it. Predictably, all of this drives decisions about the future. Entrepreneurs and inventors put more effort into developing new technologies, investors are more willing to finance these efforts, and medical students are more inclined toward the extra training needed to garner technology's rich rewards. And once these actors have placed their bets, they're motivated to play the political system to safeguard their wagers—by opposing payment cuts and other policy changes that might break the technology-reinforcing cycle.

But break it we must, in selective fashion, by rewarding decisive, high-value clinical advances while discouraging development of costly treatments that yield doubtful benefits. Transforming incentives in this way won't *reduce* medical spending,[25] but it will slow its rise. It will change the calculus of clinical investment, reducing the expected payoffs from technologies that dazzle but deliver only marginal results.

Even so, medicine's capabilities and costs will inexorably grow. Increasingly, doctors will need to say no to care that's technologically possible and that could prolong life, but that does so in competition with other national priorities. We must empower them to do so even when the consequences seem tragic. But we must give them this power without asking them to break faith at the bedside. To this end, the current regime of covert rationing, under cover of "medical necessity," should be supplanted by visible resource allocation rules—rules set for doctors and patients by social institutions. These rules will at times result in heartrending outcomes. But patients and their families will be able to see that these outcomes are the product of decisions that apply broadly. Sadness and anger will forever be part of clinical limit-setting. Betrayal at the bedside, though, can be avoided.

Largely, that is, but not entirely. At the interstices between the rules, doctors will make individualized judgments about allocation of life-prolonging resources. Amidst the competing pressures of a crowded, big-city ER, Yanira's doctors judged her report of right-side weakness insufficient to trigger a protocol that required a head CT scan if they found such weakness on physical exam. They made judgment calls about whether the rule applied and about whether to perform a more detailed clinical exam to investigate what she told them. Application of any rule or protocol requires triggering judgments—judgments about whether criteria have been met and which rule to apply.[26] Physicians ought to make these judgments with a Hippocratic bias, in favor of their patients' hopes and needs. They should be advocates, not impartial arbiters of conflict between their patients' interests and insurers' financial goals. But doctors and their patients need to acknowledge that conservation of resources is part of the picture. Just as attorneys aren't allowed to make arguments that lack a plausible basis,[27] physicians mustn't resort to outlandish interpretation to escape the meaning of rules that constrain their spending.

Physician advocacy along these lines will put pressure on health care payers to be clear about the clinical limits they mean to set. Insurers that employ vague contract terms to veil health care rationing will be stymied by physicians' exploitation of ambiguity on their patients' behalf. Clarity about clinical limits could take many forms, from cost-benefit trade-off formulas (for example, maximum expenditures on care per life-year saved) to exclusion of particular tests and treatments. What's important is that payers be up front about the reality of limits—and about the principles they employ to set them.[28]

Transparency of this sort will compel *us* to come to terms with the truth that insurers must say no to beneficial care to stay within the limits *we* impose when we seek low prices for products and services, elect politicians who promise low taxes, and choose cheaper health plans for ourselves. "Quiet hypocrisy" about health care rationing shields *us* from the contradiction between these limits and our expectation that doctors do everything.

How these limits should be set is a question for our politics. Americans with a more progressive bent will incline toward cost-benefit trade-off principles applicable to all, or at least to most of us, whether we're insured by private or government-sponsored plans. How doctors, hospitals, and insurers value our lives, many hold, should be decoupled from the existing distribution of wealth.[29] A public agency, insulated from the importunings of stakeholders, could craft cost-benefit trade-off principles, then translate them into clinical protocols for payers and providers.[30]

More market-oriented thinkers will tend to reject such "one-size-fits-all" protocols in favor of resource allocation rules specified in health plan contracts.[31] They embrace a "health care supermarket" ideal, in which people pick and choose from among cost-benefit trade-off principles, based on their ability and willingness to pay. (About this, I'll have more to say in chapter 5.) My own leanings are against tying health care tightly to economic privilege. Wealth will find ways to be served, whether through amenities like concierge floors in hospitals or by taking high-tech, rescue-oriented care to extremes. But resource allocation rules worthy of our aspirations toward fairness and equal opportunity should ensure that *all* have ready access to high-value care that promotes health, cures illness, and ameliorates suffering when cure is out of reach.

Our politics will answer these questions. Some, maybe myself included, won't like the answers. My larger point, though, is that limit-setting must be done in the open, whether through public or market means. Doing so will make *us* more active participants in priority-setting, giving patients and their families at least some sense of ownership in decisions to say no, even when the consequences are tragic. And it will free our doctors from the work of "quiet hypocrisy," work that arouses our sense of betrayal when we catch doctors doing it. We're putting growing pressure on them to do this work as medicine's costs and capabilities (and our therapeutic expectations) rise. It's a task at odds with our need for doctors to stand by us at the bedside, and it's a task that's putting trust in medicine at rising risk.

chapter four

politics, morals, and medical need I

PTSD

"We Got Him"

66 **S**ome of my family call me a ghost. I can sneak up on them." In the
service of his country, Jeans Cruz learned to kill quietly, snapping
necks and slitting throats. "Before I went to the service," he recalled when
we met in a Manhattan hotel, "I lived in a war zone—gang fights, murders,
suicides." After 9/11, he volunteered for another, enlisting in the U.S. Army
as a cavalry scout. There were ample opportunities for derring-do. Despite
disciplinary problems—"I have a short fuse," he told me—he was picked
for an elite reconnaissance team, and he rode to Baghdad, then Tikrit, in
the Iraq War's early weeks. Cruz manned the 50-caliber gunner's slot atop
a Humvee, spotting snipers and getting lucky when bullets ricocheted his
way. Men died when he saw their muzzle flashes and returned their fire with
precision. The Bronx street brawler had become a warrior, winning medals
for valor and inspiring his fellow soldiers' awe.

Cruz spent time with the "Iraq Survey Group," a euphemism for the
team tasked to look for the weapons of mass destruction that weren't found.
He was then assigned to a special forces squad charged with seizing suspected

insurgents and finding fellow soldiers taken hostage. There were more of these, he says, than the media ever reported. "Lots of our soldiers were captured. . . . They'd cut our guys' heads off. And the things we did—they were not in the press—the Geneva Conventions were crap."

As a hunter of men, Cruz excelled. "I loved working with special forces," he told me. "They were smarter—they trusted you when you showed you could do something." What he could do was to move by stealth, stay hidden in grass and trees, and quietly dispense with any locals unfortunate enough to spot him lying in wait. Dressed as a farmer, he'd sometimes walk into unfriendly villages, knowing that discovery, by a kid or a barking dog, could mean quick, violent death. More than once, he spent nights on roofs, frozen in place to keep from making a sound, listening to the conversations below.

For a week in December 2003, he was assigned to watch comings and goings at a farm on the Tigris River, near the village of Adwar. He hid in palm groves and lemon orchards, amidst swarming insurgents in Iraq's Sunni heartland. Then, on December 14, the command came to go in. A raiding party of several hundred assembled at dusk—special forces teams, scouts, and regular infantry, ignorant about the mission's objectives. "Different groups took different areas—you get instructions to cover an area. We know where the house is, where the farm is, where the water flows through. We can look at the pictures and know where they are on the map."

"We started the raid at midnight," Cruz recalled. "We went in hard. They were firing—flash, bang. Six children were in the house—most of them girls—and two wives of the owner. He didn't want to put up a fight because he didn't want his kids to be harmed. I do believe it was his brothers who were doing the shooting." Beneath the house, the raiders found tunnels and bunkers with weapons and money. The original plan had been for Cruz to ride in on a truck, as part of the strike on the main house. But plans changed. Cruz and two of his recon buddies were given an area outside the house and ordered to go in on foot, over ground thought to be booby-trapped with explosives.

Wearing night-vision gear, the three moved in, spotting landmarks they'd seen in photos and looking for wires sticking up above ground. They came across three depressions in the earth, obviously dug by human hands. Each appeared to be bomb-free. Then they noticed a small stream, not on their map, with a few PVC pipes poking up beside it. Near the pipes was a tiny foot rug, covered in mud. One of the three—Cruz doesn't recall who—lifted the rug. Beneath it was what looked like a large cinderblock, about a foot square, with ropes attached. The three pulled hard on the ropes, and the block came up easily. It was Styrofoam. Below was blackness—they'd come across an entrance to an underground space.

For a second, there was silence—and sheer terror. Then Cruz took a deadly risk. He tossed in a flash grenade, a device designed to explode in non-lethal fashion, leaving enemy personnel temporarily blind, deaf, and disoriented. "If the flash grenade had blown up other explosives, we'd have been blown up," he told me. Explosives had been found in nearby bunkers. But a second, then two, then three went by after the grenade ignited, without a follow-on blast or any other sound. To fit through the opening, Cruz took off his equipment—his pack, first-aid kit, and other strapped-on gear. He then leapt in, stumbling, then regaining his footing at the bottom of a chamber not much bigger than a powder room. A dazed and stinking man stood his ground, by a bunk bed, holding an AK-47 and a pistol.

"My heart was pumping," Cruz told me. "The guy could have fired off some rounds. I rushed him, tackled him, and got the weapons from him. All he said to us was he was the president of Iraq and he was Saddam Hussein."

"We got him out, transported him to the house, and waited for the chopper to come" to take him. "I walked back to the Humvee—my God, I thought, just let it be him so we could go home. My son, born in May—I hadn't yet seen him."

"Ladies and gentlemen, we got him," America's viceroy in Baghdad, Paul Bremer, told the world the next day. The same day, Cruz's commanders told his recon unit that their tour was being extended for several months; the insurgency was to blame. "We had a week off [after capturing Saddam], then we went back on missions. Because we were requested. You know what—I feel honored to be requested. But God damn, give me a break."

Just two weeks after taking Saddam, Cruz returned from a combat operation soaked in blood from a wounded comrade. Within hours, he was on his way to Baghdad, then to Baltimore-Washington airport, for some time with his family. "I'd just got back from a mission—for five days straight, I didn't have a shower. The guys gave me some money to fly to New York—my friends gave me $400.[1] I was still wearing the bloody uniform on the flight from Baltimore to LaGuardia."

Memories

Cruz came home to his wife, infant son, and American-style celebrity. Appearances on ABC's *The View*, CNN with Paula Zahn, and other programs followed. He was suddenly one of the county's most celebrated soldiers— an icon of post-9/11 patriotism and derring-do. Then it was back to Iraq's Sunni heartland and combat's random terror. And his resilience began to falter. "You start having hallucinations—a tank, when there's nothing there. Our commanders would say it's from the heat." There were nightmares and panic attacks—and an altercation with an officer. Cruz had been promoted from specialist to sergeant, but then, he recalled, "a new guy took over our unit—a West Point grad, a captain—they get into your face. He grabbed me. I pushed him and put him in a chokehold. He was disciplined, and I was demoted."

His body took a battering as well. A month or so before Saddam's capture, Cruz had gone on a mission that involved some rock climbing. "The guy in front of me got scared by a bat and let go of the rope. I fell twenty feet. My rucksack frame hit my kidneys. There was blood in my urine. My back hurt—severe pains and constant spasms." The back pains and bloody urine never went away. On another recon mission, his unit began taking mortar fire. "We started running. There were small holes [in the ground]. I fell—my foot slipped down the side of a hole. I got up and kept running." Only after they'd escaped did he notice the swelling and pain. And a year went by before doctors found that he'd fractured bones in his foot and that they'd grown together the wrong way.

Memories pursued him relentlessly through the night. "On September 18, 2003, we were ambushed from both sides by fifty to sixty guys. There were thirteen of us. They hit us hard, from RPGs [rocket-propelled grenades] to AKs [AK-47s] to little fireballs—pure hell. There were guys trying to run, and guys just dropping. That was really hard." Another time, he recalled, "They gave me a new guy" to look out for—a fresh arrival without combat experience. "Then the commander sent him to another point. I said, 'What are you doing with my soldier—he's my responsibility.'" Jeans then pointed to the back of his head to show what happened minutes later. "The bullet entered here and went out through his forehead. Thirteen hours before, we were talking—he talked to me about his new marriage, wife, and child. . . . I wrote her a letter."

There are uglier memories, even more relentless. "There were certain missions where we had to keep everything quiet." But sometimes, he told me, they'd encounter children while hiding in trees, on roofs, or elsewhere. The kids, he said, would set off a ruckus, revealing the Americans' positions. Some special forces commanders claimed the kids didn't do so innocently. Insurgents, they said, sent kids out to look for U.S. troops and to make noise so their fighters could flee—or attack—when the Americans appeared. The preventive measure practiced by special forces soldiers on stealth missions, Cruz said, was to silence anyone who might out them, by killing quietly if need be.

The memories, for Cruz, are agonizing and recurrent. They force themselves upon him at unpredictable moments—when he sees children playing on the South Bronx streets or when he looks into his six-year-old son's eyes. "I think of those kids . . . Most of the times we just held the kids. . . . Once or twice, a kid—three, four, or five years old"—he paused—"the things we did . . . I held them 'til—one or two times"—he paused again, then said he slit their throats.

There've been claims that special forces soldiers in Iraq ran wild as they went after insurgents and that high-level commanders sanctioned the sort of behavior Cruz described. There've been no mainstream media confirmations; nor could Cruz name places, people, or fighting units involved. From the perspective of personal accountability and rule-of-law, the veracity of these claims matters enormously. The acts Cruz describes are, of course, war crimes. But from the perspective of Cruz's mental health, whether his crimes are real or imagined may matter much less. What's clear is that Cruz *believes* he did these things and that the beliefs permit him no peace.

In March 2004, Cruz's tour of duty in Iraq came to an end. He'd not see combat again. With most of the Fourth Infantry, he was airlifted to Fort Hood, Texas, the division's home. His life deteriorated from there. The nightmares and panic attacks grew worse. He developed asthma that kept him out of training maneuvers, and his relationship with his wife fell apart. He was permitted to re-enlist but sent to psychological counseling. The therapeutic relationship didn't quite work out. His psychiatrist—he remembers her only as "Dr. Gray, a short black woman"—didn't listen, he told me, and that made him mad. "She said 'uh-huh' a lot. One time, I got up, and I yelled at her because she wasn't paying attention. . . . I tried saying some real stupid stuff to see if she noticed. Like, 'I murdered this girl. Oh, I killed somebody the other day because she was laughing.'"

Things got worse. There were more altercations—with officers, fellow soldiers, and medical personnel. "I ended up being attacked by six MPs [military police] because I started fighting," he recalled, "throwing tables and chairs." Groups of people bothered him. "Crowds set me off. I feared someone will start shooting and there'll be nowhere to run. . . . I can't be around more than two or three people."

Cruz was experiencing the classic symptoms of posttraumatic stress disorder, or PTSD, a psychiatric diagnosis crafted in the 1970s and 1980s to capture the experience of thousands of Vietnam veterans. War trauma has an ancient history. Accounts of it date back to classical Greece, though the greater intensity of mechanized combat with high explosives has made battle more psychologically devastating over the past hundred years. "Shell shock," "war neurosis," and "battle fatigue" are among the other terms variously invoked since World War I's devastating psychic toll brought the problem to clinical prominence. Historians of medicine who have studied clinical thinking about war trauma since the Civil and Crimean wars have found wide fluctuations in symptoms recorded and ideas about the illness.[2] But at the core of the concept of PTSD since the Vietnam era have been three "clusters" of symptoms: (1) intrusive recall of a traumatic moment, often through nightmares or flashbacks, (2) avoidance of thoughts and activities associated with a traumatic experience (often accompanied by numbing of emotions and by feelings of estrangement from others), and (3) increased arousal (including irritability, sleep difficulties, and inability to concentrate).[3] Cruz experienced multiple symptoms within each of these clusters.

Politics

Cruz's symptoms qualified him for the diagnosis of PTSD, as defined by the source that doctors, health insurers, and the armed services treat as authoritative. That source, the American Psychiatric Association's *Diagnostic and Statistical Manual of Mental Disorders, Fourth Edition* (*DSM-4-TR*[4]), is one of psychiatry's great success stories. Before 1980, psychiatrists lacked generally accepted standards for the diagnosis of mental illnesses. Their professional association maintained a diagnostic manual, but its disease categories were vaguely defined and based on controversial theories about the origin or course of mental illnesses. Psychiatrists often ignored its disease definitions or applied them inconsistently. The result was skepticism about what psychiatry had to offer—and reluctance by health insurers to pay for it.

In the late 1970s, the profession's leaders took action. The American Psychiatric Association (APA) set about developing a diagnostic scheme disconnected from arguments over the etiology of mental illnesses and based on standardized, easy-to-apply criteria. Committees of psychiatrists reached agreement on dozens of diagnostic constructs, including PTSD. This unity has held since, through three revisions of the diagnostic manual that embodied it.[5]

Health insurers and public agencies that provide medical care (including the Pentagon and the U.S. Department of Veterans Affairs [VA]) have adopted the APA manual's diagnostic categories and criteria. As a psychiatrist in training in the late 1980s, I was taught that these categories and criteria were the product of science—epidemiological studies showing that these disorders existed. The criteria for PTSD, I learned, followed from state-of-the-art understanding of war trauma[6] and its psychic effects. Neither politics nor moral judgment played any role; PTSD and its criteria represented psychiatry's best effort to describe a syndrome found in nature. But as Jeans Cruz underwent evaluation for his intrusive memories and explosive behavior, a political challenge to the diagnosis of PTSD was in full swing.

Right-wing critics of the diagnosis claimed it miscasts personal challenge as pathological process.[7] The horrors of war, they said, call for courage and resilience, not the makeover of warriors as victims. Men and women who return home from combat must reconcile their battlefield experiences with their lives before and after. This challenge calls for character, not the dependence that accompanies the "sick" role, critics held. The culture of therapy, they argued, rewards passivity, not personal responsibility. It coddles dysfunction and punishes self-reliance by withholding free health care and disability benefits from those who don't prevail upon their doctors to diagnose PTSD. More insidiously, PTSD's conservative critics complained, it gives short shrift to armed conflict as an honorable endeavor by encouraging citizens to stigmatize its veterans as sufferers, not heroes.

This challenge began well before the wars spawned by 9/11. In the late 1990s, Vietnam veterans' claims for medical care and disability for delayed-onset PTSD soared,[8] arousing the ire of PTSD-skeptics. Tying health and disability benefits to decades-old traumatic memories, the skeptics said, discouraged veterans from taking responsibility for their own lives. Military action in Iraq charged the PTSD debate with new meaning. "It has become a pro-war versus anti-war issue," a VA official told the *Washington Post* (on condition of anonymity) in 2005. "If we show that PTSD is prevalent and severe, that becomes one more little reason we should stop waging war. If, on the other hand, PTSD rates are low . . . that is convenient for the Bush Administration."[9]

As America's engagement in Iraq deepened, the politics of PTSD took on a higher profile. Independent surveys of the disorder's incidence among Iraq War veterans yielded estimates as high as 20 percent.[10] The Pentagon's own study of mental illness among Iraq and Afghanistan veterans found that 15 to 20 percent of troops fighting in the two conflicts showed signs of depression or PTSD, and that this figure rose to 30 percent for soldiers on their third or forth combat deployment.[11] Critics of the war—and of the Pentagon's stewardship of strategy and tactics—charged the Bush administration with understating the conflict's human and financial costs.[12] Thanks to technological advances and speedy medical evacuation, military doctors achieved unprecedented success at saving lives.[13] For every American killed in action in Iraq as of September 30, 2006, eight wounded soldiers survived, an astonishing improvement over the ratios of 2.6 wounded per fatality in Vietnam, 2.8 in Korea, and 1.6 in World War II.[14] But more survivors meant more veterans with lifelong clinical needs—and higher long-term costs for American taxpayers. Along with traumatic brain injury and major depression, PTSD emerged as one of the war's signature health consequences.

Battles over how many billions of dollars these consequences would cost ensued. So did charges that the Bush administration was neglecting the needs of traumatized veterans—by putting them through multiple tours of combat duty without sufficient respite and by failing to provide them with the medical care and social support they urgently needed. Estimates of the lifetime costs of providing health care and disability benefits to the Iraq war's wounded and traumatized veterans ranged as high as $700 billion.[15] Democrats in Congress condemned the administration's failure to budget for war's mental health burden. Veterans' advocates complained about long queues for care and failure to provide state-of-the-art treatment.

The Bush administration pushed back, targeting PTSD. Amid reports of internal pressure on military and VA clinicians to diagnose PTSD less frequently, the administration lobbied American psychiatry's powers that be to demedicalize the aftereffects of combat by narrowing the criteria for the diagnosis. Administration officials even tried an end run around the APA by urging the Institute of Medicine, an affiliate of the National Academies of Sciences, to revisit the rules for diagnosing PTSD.

In support of this effort, PTSD skeptics could point to some science. Studies of the incidence of PTSD *symptoms* and of traumatic events serious enough to "count" for the purpose of diagnosing the disorder (the diagnosis requires both the requisite symptoms and a past traumatic experience) found little or no correlation between the two.[16] An examination of depressed patients found that they were equally likely to satisfy symptom checklists for PTSD whether or not they experienced *trauma* sufficient to qualify. This, the skeptics said, showed that the symptoms were caused by something other than psychic trauma. PTSD thus made no sense as a diagnostic entity, they argued, since it presumed a causal connection (between trauma and symptoms) that didn't exist.

But the campaign against PTSD failed to sway psychiatry's leaders. Not only did the APA stand by its broad definition; the Institute of Medicine twice reaffirmed it. In two reports, one commissioned by the VA with the express aim of reducing PTSD-related health spending, the Institute backed the APA's approach. This was hardly a surprise. The Institute develops its policy recommendations by appointing panels of experts, typically drawn from the upper reaches of medical academia, clinical practice, and health policy. The panels appointed to weigh PTSD were chosen from psychiatry's elite, the same pool of researchers and clinicians tapped to draft the APA's diagnostic manual. For conservative critics of PTSD, this was proof that the fix was on: American psychiatry's elite was using its institutional perches to protect a diagnostic construct that promoted practitioners' economic interests, unduly burdened taxpayers, and patronized veterans by treating them as victims.

Diagnosis and Discretion

Within the military and the VA, resistance continued out of public view. Army doctors have told me of ongoing pressure to keep PTSD diagnoses to a minimum. From the Pentagon's perspective, the stakes are enormous. Findings that up to a fifth of those who served in Iraq developed PTSD (and that a third or more of all Iraq and Afghanistan veterans eventually met the APA's diagnostic criteria for one or another serious mental illness)[17] raised alarm about the devastating effect that diagnosis of PTSD and other psychiatric disorders could have on military manpower. And that's not to mention the costs of long-term mental health care and disability pay for these psychiatric casualties of war.

The army's covert campaign against PTSD has flashed into view from time to time, as when, in June 2008, a soldier secretly taped his psychologist's admission that "all the clinicians up here are being pressured to not diagnose PTSD."[18] (The psychologist, Douglas McNinch, said he was urged to employ a different diagnosis, "anxiety disorder not otherwise specified," not caused by combat stress.) A year earlier, the *Army Times* and *NPR* reported that a psychiatrist picked by the army's medical command to review dozens of disputed diagnoses (cases in which army doctors attributed soldiers' post-combat problems to character flaws rather than PTSD or brain injury) had in fact *made* or *overseen* these diagnoses as chief of behavioral health at Fort Carson, Colorado.[19] The psychiatrist, Colonel Steven Knorr, explained to an interviewer that battle stress can bring out previously unnoticed, life-long personality problems.[20] "We have to hold Soldiers accountable for their behavior," Knorr wrote in a memo to his clinical staff, obtained by *NPR*'s Daniel Zwerdling. "Everyone in life beyond babies, the insane, and the de-mented and mentally retarded [*sic*] have to be held accountable for what they do in life."

In May 2008, a veterans' group critical of the Bush administration's Iraq policies released an e-mail it obtained, from a VA psychologist in Texas to her staff, putting the brakes on PTSD. "Given that we are having more and more compensation-seeking veterans," the psychologist, Norma Perez, wrote, "I'd like to suggest that you refrain from giving a diagnosis of PTSD straight out. Consider a diagnosis of 'adjustment disorder . . . '"[21] VA secretary James Peake quickly denied that Perez's e-mail constituted policy. It had been "re-pudiated at the highest level," he said, and Perez had been "counseled." But the media kerfuffle over the episode brought attention to another senior VA official's comments a few months earlier, when queried in court about whether the department was downplaying battle stress. Under questioning in a class action suit alleging VA neglect of former soldiers' psychiatric prob-lems, the agency's undersecretary for health, Dr. Michael Kussman, insisted:

"It is unfair and inappropriate to stigmatize people with a mental health di-agnosis when they are having what most people believe are normal reactions to an abnormal situation."

Jeans Cruz's psychiatrist at Fort Hood, Lieutenant Colonel Sharette Gray, evaluated him against the backdrop of the rising controversy over PTSD. She and the others responsible for his health care found symptoms of anxiety and depression, including nightmares, and prescribed mood-stabilizing drugs to manage them. Other doctors would later conclude that Cruz had the symp-toms to qualify for a PTSD diagnosis. But instead of conferring this diagno-sis, Dr. Gray recorded a finding of "personality disorder" and recommended Cruz's immediate discharge from the army. Cruz's commanding officers as-sented, and he was mustered out against his will[22]—less than six months after he'd re-enlisted. More than that, he was denied medical and disability benefits.[23] Cruz's "personality disorder" was the army's equivalent of a health plan member's "pre-existing condition"—carte blanche to deny benefits on the ground that his "disorder" predated his 2002 army enlistment.

It got worse. "My wife 5–13'd me," he recalled—a wry reference to the regulation that permitted Dr. Gray and his superiors to force him out. And as his marriage failed, the army froze his bank account to recoup his $10,000 re-enlistment bonus. Cruz's car was repossessed—he couldn't make the pay-ments. In June 2005, three weeks after his discharge, the couple joined the ranks of America's homeless. No cable news crew covered their forced depar-ture from the residence the Fourth Infantry provided at Fort Hood. "I had to sleep in a U-Haul with my wife for two days."

The couple returned to the Bronx, then went their separate ways. Cruz—by now in a wheelchair, with chronic back and leg pain, continuing asthma attacks, and blood in his urine from his mysterious kidney injury—lost custody of his older son. He moved in with his parents but was unable to get medical coverage. And the VA wouldn't treat him even for problems, like his back and kidney ailments, plainly due to the beating his body took in Iraq. In theory, he was eligible since these were "service-connected" condi-tions. But the "personality disorder" discharge had pushed him into a bu-reaucratic black hole. It had forced him out before an army medical board could approve him for care from the VA. He could apply to the VA on his own, but he'd be placed at the back of a queue that might take years. Had army medical reviewers approved him, he could have obtained care from the VA right away.

Cruz also struggled to get a grip on his explosive reactions to things he saw in civilian life that rubbed him the wrong way. "Coming out of the service, I wanted to relax, but people kept pushing my buttons," he said. "My sister walks around cursing. What kind of culture is it? . . . Nowadays you hit a kid with a belt and he wants to call the cops on you." The pressure inside built, and there was nowhere, no way, to let it out. "My training makes me feel above everybody else—discipline, character, state of mind. . . . People's stupidity—that sets me off now. If your common sense isn't like someone else's common sense, and you make the mistake of physically or emotionally hurting somebody, then I don't tolerate that." He became aggravated on crowded streets, when people talked loudly or cut in front of him. And he endured more intimate humiliation—loss of bladder control that forced him to wear an adult diaper. And from his wheelchair, he couldn't be the father he expected himself to be. "My son—it's 'Daddy, let's play football, let's play basketball.' Daddy can't do all those things."

It's easy to admonish Dr. Gray for her "personality disorder" diagnosis—and to condemn the Bush administration for politicizing the diagnosis of PTSD to downplay the cost of a controversial war. Veterans' groups and members of Congress have done so for understandable reasons: There's mounting evidence that thousands of Iraq and Afghanistan veterans are suffering from combat stress that hasn't been recognized by the armed services or the VA. But to claim that the concept of PTSD is *apolitical* is to ignore the cultural and moral choices embedded in both the APA's definition of the disorder and the definition's application to Cruz and others.

Any grouping of people's behaviors and experiences for the purpose of medical diagnosis makes a cultural and moral statement—one that stresses biological determinants and thus discounts people's power to shape their lives. Diagnosis confers forgiveness at the price of moral passivity. When behaviors and experiences become signs and symptoms, society refrains from conferring credit or blame. This is not to say that the disempowerment associated with diagnosis precludes all judgment about character. Patients can show courage, even heroism, by enduring uncertainty, suffering, and awareness of a dismal clinical fate. They can do so through their quiet dignity and loving concern for others. By so doing, they can affirm a measure of authorship over their lives. But disease calls for deference to doctors and compliance with their treatments. Thus diagnosis shrinks the possibilities for displaying character. This has been the case since the Hippocratics recast diseases as naturalistic phenomena rather than evidence of one's being out of sorts with the gods.

So to say that the anxieties and agitation of former combatants constitute disease is to make a statement about the scope of their personal responsibility. It's also to issue a declaration about the *state's* responsibility, since the state sent them to war, exposing them to battle stress and its biological consequences. That moral judgments are embedded in the definition of PTSD is underscored by the APA manual's lack of disease categories corresponding to other life challenges. No APA "disorders" mobilize health insurers to pay for SAT prep courses after poor test scores, mentors for troubled underclass kids, marriage counselors for relationships torn asunder by job stress, or sexual surrogates for men and women ill at ease with erotic intimacy. What is "medical" is a moral and cultural matter. Most Americans treat personal accomplishment—in the workplace and at home and school—as a matter of individual responsibility. And they view erotic experience as something that shouldn't be sold for a price.[24] The APA manual incorporates this moral outlook. Doctors who apply the manual to their patients are thus agents of public morality, whether or not they're consciously aware of it.

They are, in this sense, *political* actors, with a small "p," ratifying and reinforcing moral precepts as they go about their Hippocratic duties. More than that, they expound upon the APA manual's embedded moral outlook as they apply its diagnostic criteria, case by case. Like judges who give meaning to a statute by construing it in myriad circumstances, they interpret the manual's criteria as they assess each patient. The manual's definition of "traumatic" experience, a prerequisite for PTSD, isn't mathematically precise. It compels clinicians to make a series of subjective judgments—about whether an event "involved . . . threatened death or serious injury," whether a patient "experienced, witnessed, or was confronted with" such an event, and whether his or her "response involved intense fear, helplessness, or horror."

Since combat, by its very nature, means being the object of the enemy's lethal endeavors, this definition could well apply to everyone in the line of fire. In a fight against insurgents, moreover, the boundary lines of combat dissolve. All are potential targets—of secreted explosive devices, stray mortar shells, and other efforts to kill and maim. So, in theory, just about anyone in theater, in Iraq or Afghanistan, could qualify for the definition. All face *some* threat of death or injury; to not feel afraid requires a fair measure of denial. To narrow the range of traumatic experiences that permit diagnosis—to include fewer than *all*—doctors must exercise some interpretive restraint. The sinews for this restraint are moral beliefs about the danger and fear that fighting men and women *ought* to be able to endure.

The APA manual's other criteria for PTSD are no less open to field discretion. Its checklists for assessment of the several PTSD symptom "clusters" call for subjective judgments about such things as the intrusiveness of bad memories, loss of hope for the future, and levels of irritability and anger. The manual also requires doctors to make a call as to whether a patient's "disturbance" (i.e., "symptoms," taken as a whole) "causes clinically significant distress and/or impairment in social, occupational, and/or other important areas of functioning." But life deals out disappointment to us all: The happily married, Nobel Prize-winning CEOs (with kids at Harvard) among us are few. So, unless all deficits of personal fulfillment are to be deemed "clinically significant" (great for psychotherapists but bad news for health insurers), doctors must make *moral* judgments about the degree of "distress" and "impairment" that people should be expected to endure.

Like judges who rely on rules announced in prior court opinions, clinicians cabin their personal discretion by looking to guidance from professional leaders and to the practices of their peers. That's what Dr. Gray did when confronted with Jeans Cruz's complex history—distressing experiences and behavior that powerfully suggested PTSD, predated by a "short fuse" on the Bronx's mean streets and a defiant attitude toward superiors during basic training. His insolence may well have been key to survival on the urban street. But his explosive behavior before and after he first saw combat raised the possibility of borderline personality disorder. His self-mutilating acts, including slashing his forearms and burning himself with cigarettes, are classic borderline personality features. And his brushes with the law (and with commanding officers) suggested antisocial personality disorder.

What, if anything, army medical leaders said to Dr. Gray by way of guidance remains a mystery, about which the military will say little.[25] But there have been numerous reports of importunings to clinicians to emphasize soldiers' pre-deployment life difficulties and to take a skeptical stance toward their accounts of combat exposure. Dr. Gray did both. Her conclusion that Cruz had a long-standing personality disorder rested on his pre-enlistment troubles, rage attacks, and refusals to follow orders. Remarkably, moreover, Gray didn't credit Cruz with having experienced enough stress to qualify for PTSD—despite awards for valor and worldwide recognition for his leap into Saddam Hussein's bunker.

Politics Over Science?

After he returned to New York, Cruz sought help from the Bronx VA Medical Center. Seeing his story differently, a psychologist there diagnosed PTSD and backed his VA petition for medical and disability benefits. But VA medical reviewers refused to overturn the army's diagnosis, pointing to his pre-deployment difficulties and claiming that his evidence of battle stress wasn't enough. Until Cruz lost his ability to move around on his own, he fixed boilers for a living, going without health insurance as his asthma and other health problems worsened. Then a *Washington Post* reporter, Dana Priest, learned about Cruz from veterans' health activists while researching a story about the unmet mental health needs of the men and women who'd fought in Afghanistan and Iraq. Cruz's story led her piece, which ran on page 1, almost exactly two years after he was forced from his home at Fort Hood.

Within four days, thirty-one Senators had written to Defense Secretary Robert Gates to call for an inquiry into abuse of "personality disorder" discharges and to urge "appropriate measures to prevent the repeat of cases like Specialist Cruz's . . . ."[26] Republican senator Kit Bond (MO) charged that Cruz and others given this diagnosis were being "railroaded,"[27] Democrat Barack Obama introduced a bill to freeze "personality disorder" discharges pending an inquiry, and most of the major TV news networks ran segments spotlighting Cruz and others affected. Grammy Award winner Dave Matthews seized on the issue, telling a Radio City Music Hall audience that the case of another wounded soldier discharged for a "personality disorder," Jon Town, was an "injustice so blatant that it just makes you feel like you're gonna die of sorrow."[28] Matthews denounced the practice again on ABC News's *This Week.* A House committee held hearings. Commentators and legislators queued up to condemn the "personality disorder" discharge as a sham.

In January 2008, President Bush signed legislation requiring the Defense Department to report on its "personality disorder" discharge procedures, including precautions taken to ensure that men and women suffering from PTSD and other combat-related conditions aren't cashiered on "personality disorder" grounds. The Pentagon responded by denying the problem, concluding that "[t]here is no indication that personality disorder diagnoses for members who were deployed in support of the Global War on Terror were prone to systematic or widespread error."[29] But the army and the VA reversed their decisions on Jeans Cruz, granting him a diagnosis of PTSD. He became eligible for care from the Bronx VA for his array of medical and mental health problems.

For veterans' advocates—and for the thirty-one senators who signed the letter to Gates—this result was a victory for proper diagnosis over Pentagon politics. For PTSD skeptics, it was a triumph of politics over science. Research showing little or no correlation between PTSD *symptoms* and the traumatic exposure needed to qualify for the diagnosis is consistent with Knorr's claim that battle stress brings out previously unnoticed personality disorders. We vary enormously in our abilities to adapt to stressors large and small. Traumatic experiences that aren't bad enough to qualify for PTSD (which, as defined by the APA, requires exposure to intense stress) can trigger PTSD *symptoms* in many people. This is particularly likely in people who meet APA criteria for personality disorders. Conversely, many (probably most) people who experience trauma serious enough to qualify for PTSD don't develop the symptoms needed to diagnose it. They're resilient enough to adapt.

PTSD skeptics like Knorr point to this as reason for doubt when soldiers present with PTSD symptoms. In the APA manual, they note, some of these symptoms do double duty as diagnostic criteria for both PTSD and personality disorders. The manual requires clinicians to make judgment calls.

Clinical judgments—and the spending that accompanies them—are much influenced by moral and cultural politics. In the wrangling over whether the Pentagon and the VA underdiagnosed PTSD, both sides claimed clinical science supported them. Each cast the other as disingenuous. But science couldn't answer the questions they contested. The army's critics, in my view, had the weight of clinical *opinion* on their side. Surely being shot at, watching a buddy die, or even traveling on roads mined with IEDs [improvised explosive devices] ought to "count" as trauma for PTSD purposes if exposure to school shootings or street violence suffices in civilian life; otherwise the army's approach would be inconsistent with civilian clinical practice. But embedded within civilian practice are assumptions about what people should and shouldn't be expected to endure—assumptions that impose enormous burdens on a military campaign. Diagnosing PTSD based on these premises could result in wholesale disruption of fighting units. All combat troops risk mortal wounds, many are shot at, and in warfare against insurgents who send suicide bombers into public squares, even soldiers in supporting roles are at deadly risk.

Studies indicating that up to 20 percent of soldiers came home with PTSD after one or a few Iraq deployments underline the disruptive potential of PTSD diagnosis based on prevailing clinical beliefs about what should count as trauma. Medicalization of combat experience fits awkwardly with martial virtues of grit and stoicism in the face of danger, virtues that might not maximize long-term psychic well-being but that empower men and women to keep cool while risking all for their county. And medicalization of combat memories leaves a long budgetary "tail"—a half century or more of national commitment to "care for those who shall have borne the battle."[30]

This is hardly to say that soldiers should bear these burdens by forgoing medical benefits or disability pay—or by going back into battle psychically damaged. But it is to say that competing cultural and moral beliefs—about courage, character, and who should bear the costs of combat—drive disputes over the definition and diagnosis of PTSD. And it is to say that diagnosis of PTSD is a political act—an act that affirms cultural and moral norms under cover of clinical judgment. That most psychiatrists aren't consciously aware of PTSD's political content doesn't make this any less so. But encrypting this content within the neutral-sounding language of clinical assessment stifles discussion of the political questions at stake. Neither the Institute of Medicine reports on PTSD nor the APA manual acknowledge that diagnosis incorporates cultural and moral premises and directs society's resources accordingly. Doctors think they're practicing medicine divorced from politics, on behalf of their patients, not public morals.

The Hippocratic Myth powerfully reinforces this belief. It makes separation of medical care from politics an ethical obligation. It thus turns candor about the political balances embedded in PTSD diagnosis into an ethical embarrassment for physicians. But these political judgments are a public matter. The balance between therapeutic compassion and the martial virtues of grit and stoicism, the extent of the sacrifice we should expect from men and women who face mortal danger on our behalf, and the matter of what we owe them in return are questions for democratic decision. They deserve searching discussion by citizens and elected leaders. We shouldn't defer to the drafters of diagnostic criteria to resolve these questions furtively. Only by recognizing that diagnosis is a political act—an act that advances cultural and moral values—can we engage citizens in the pursuit of answers.

chapter five

politics, morals, and medical need II

mobilizing shared resources

*A*ll medical diagnosis is political. It defines personal characteristics—signs and symptoms—as both undesirable ("pathological") and beyond the scope of one's own responsibility. To be sure, some diagnoses suggest a measure of before-the-fact culpability: think lung cancer and smoking or HIV infection and reckless sex. Likewise, compliance with treatment is a matter of personal responsibility: We take a dim view of tuberculosis patients who stop their antibiotics or diabetics who don't control their blood sugar. But once an illness is named and blamed, *it* becomes a culpable agent—the common foe of doctor and patient. Diagnosis mobilizes social resources (public and private insurance) for the fight, and it excuses people from myriad social obligations.

Because the political content of most diagnoses isn't controversial, we tend not to give it much thought. We don't debate whether pneumococcal pneumonia is an illness, and we don't much quibble over its diagnostic criteria—shortness of breath, a scary-looking chest X-ray, and proof that pneumococci are present. In a trivial sense, though, we're making a political choice. From the pneumococci's point of view, lungs are a nice place to feed and multiply, and taking their lives with antibiotics is a nasty thing.

Fortunately, doctors aren't bedeviled by bacterial rights activists; they kill to cure, and we (and our insurers) are willing to pay them for it. We're happy, also, to treat heart attacks and strokes as diseases—and to take pricey measures to save people who suffer them. No one complains that doing so keeps people around past their appointed time.

What's a Disease?

But more disease constructs than we might imagine incorporate contestable cultural and moral premises. This is least surprising in psychiatry. Many of the diagnoses in the APA's manual of mental disorders rest on subjective beliefs about what we ought to aspire to in life and how we should respond to challenges and disappointments. Consider "adjustment disorder," a box commonly checked by clinicians seeking insurance payment for outpatient psychotherapy. This diagnosis turns on subjective impressions of the degree of distress that's to be "expected" after a romantic breakup, job loss, or other painful event (distress "in excess" of what's expected qualifies for the diagnosis—and for coverage).[1] But beliefs about what *should* be "expected" vary. It's the stuff of cliché that emotive Italians and reticent English differ in their responses to failed romance and life's other disappointments. The clichés may be overwrought, but there are cultural differences in how people react to life's troubles—differences that translate into varied takes on the distress that's "expected." A clinician can't diagnose adjustment disorder without taking a position on how distraught a patient *ought* to be.

Likewise, this "disorder" requires "significant impairment in social, occupational or educational functioning."[2] Not only is this standard wide open to subjective calls about what counts as "significant impairment"; it's biased against people who aren't on life's fast track. That's because people in distress are more likely to falter in roles that require initiative and concentration than in activities that let them zone out. The CEO and the neurosurgeon will fare less well at work than a similarly troubled turnpike toll taker. Adjustment disorder is an upmarket diagnosis. It mobilizes health insurance resources more readily on behalf of the well off. From an economic efficiency perspective, this is defensible, if unappealing. Treating corporate leaders adds social value to the extent that it boosts their performance. Treating toll takers in equal distress adds nothing (beyond improvement in their well-being) so long as their distress doesn't hold them back from giving change as drivers pass through. The doctor who diagnoses adjustment disorder in the CEO but not the toll taker is an agent of this reverse Robin Hood policy. But this agency is mostly unwitting—the policy is embedded in the APA manual's rules, which don't acknowledge the distributive politics at play.

The APA manual's personality disorders, another trigger for spending on psychotherapy, rest visibly on common sense about how to go along to get along under prevailing social conditions. The criteria for narcissistic personality disorder are a catalog of behaviors and attitudes that won't win style points at the office. Such characteristics as "a grandiose sense of self-importance," "belie[f] that [one] is 'special' and unique," and "a sense of entitlement" with "unreasonable expectations of especially favorable treatment"[3] seem calculated to irritate coworkers and the boss. Employees who irk in this manner make the common pursuit of managers' objectives more difficult, or at least unpleasant. But consider, say, a midlevel executive at General Motors in 2002 who resists the push to build more SUVs, predicting a market turn toward fuel-efficient cars. When his boss insists, he can either step in line or stand firm, pointing, perhaps, to oil price predictions at odds with GM strategy. If he does the latter while his co-workers conform, he's a lone dissenter—the stuff of romantic myth (if he turns out to be right), but annoying to the boss and to others willing to go with the program.

Does he have "a grandiose sense of self-importance" (first item on the APA checklist), since he's putting himself at odds with all around him, or a belief that he's "special"? Is the answer yes if he irks his officemates, even if gas prices later soar and the market for SUVs collapses? That a psychiatrist could diagnose narcissistic personality disorder on this basis underscores the disorder's dependence on go-along-to-get-along norms of conduct.

Many of the outsized success stories in American life have been driven by "fantasies of unlimited success" (item 2 on the APA list) and "special" providence. Doris Kearns Goodwin's biography of Abraham Lincoln, *Team of Rivals,* highlights Lincoln's conviction as a twenty-something, against all odds, that he'd someday shape history. To his fellow rivercraft pilots and, later, circuit-riding lawyers, this would surely have seemed "grandiose," unless well hidden. Lincoln was "often envious of others" (diagnostic criterion 8), particularly those whose "longing to rise"[4] found satisfaction sooner than his own.

I live, most of the time, in Washington, DC, where "arrogant, haughty behaviors or attitudes" (criterion 9) are endemic among the princes and vassals of the political and policy wonk worlds. More often than I'd like to remember, I've been on the receiving end. Many try hard to "associate with other special or high-status people" (criterion 3) and "tak[e] advantage of others to achieve [their] own ends" (criterion 6). Some know few bounds, as their financial and sexual peccadilloes show. Are they narcissists? Perhaps. Research data support the conclusion that the character traits on the APA list travel together as a personal style. It's a style I find noxious. I'd like to believe a person can accomplish great things without exploiting, intimidating, and otherwise abusing underlings and peers. But whether it's a mental illness is another matter.

Treating it as such sends the message to those who aren't in life's alpha roles that such behavior isn't to be tolerated. Meanwhile, we license, even celebrate the same behavior by Donald Trump, A-Rod, and others who've established fiefdoms and command awe. Marking such self-involvement as an illness when it antagonizes the boss helps to maintain order. And diagnosis mobilizes social resources (insurance) to pursue character change. If therapy succeeds, the "sick" person becomes both happier and more productive—within society's constraints. The therapist, wittingly or otherwise, acts as an agent of these constraints.

Beyond the realm of psychiatry, contests over the political content of clinical diagnosis are more widely spaced. Nobody sides with the streptococcus in its struggle for a home in our hearts, and we turn against our own tissues when they mount cancerous insurrections. Streptococcal endocarditis and myriad malignancies are diseases by consensus because we agree on the proper response. We wage *war* on these conditions without reservation or remorse.

But consider short stature or corpulence. Well into the 1990s, parents and pediatricians considered shortness to be a trait unless caused by known illnesses—for example, intestinal malabsorption, tumors, and genetic defects. Children who were, say, among the shortest 5 percent of their age-matched peers were just little, or petite, or diminutive, not diseased. Then recombinant human growth hormone became available—as, all the while, parents became more aware of the social advantages that correlate with stature. Next, not surprisingly, came calls to treat so-called "idiopathic short stature"[5] as a disease, calls supported by companies that make growth hormone. In 2003, the Food and Drug Administration (FDA) allowed Eli Lilly to sell growth hormone as a treatment for idiopathic short stature. Three years later, a team of academics estimated the cost: $100,000, almost all of which goes to the drug maker, to add two inches to a 10-year-old boy's adult height.[6]

In its petition to the FDA, Lilly defined "short stature" restrictively: only the shortest 1.2 percent of kids qualified. But as Lilly executives knew, this opened the door to much broader, more profitable off-label use—if insurers could be persuaded to pay. Some pediatricians pushed the proposition that the shortest 5 percent should be diagnosed. Beyond the enormous cost— about $10 billion a year if the shortest 5 percent of all American children were treated at age ten—are some awkward questions. Should we tinker with our children's size to boost their job or dating prospects? If being short is a sickness, what about insufficiently pouty lips or perky breasts, or a time in the forty yard dash that's too slow to make the football coach's cut? And once we bill insurers $100,000 a shot so the shortest 5 percent can grow, what about the next 5 percent, now the shortest? At what point do we say no? We can't answer these questions without rendering judgments about rival aesthetics, public values, and what we should and shouldn't accept as fate.

Obesity is a more visible flashpoint for conflict over what constitutes disease. As I loaded my squash onto a supermarket checkout counter a while back, fretting about getting fat, four fudgy brownies vied for my attention. They looked longingly at me from the cover of *Family Circle*, distracting me for a moment from the brunette in clingy jeans on the magazine rack to the right. The cover promised that these "One-Bowl Brownies" were "fast and easy"—and that the "Super Diet" in the same issue "fights fat and boosts energy." Below the "Super Diet" on the same cover was another banner, "Best Burgers," followed by, "What Your Husband Wants You to Know about Sex." As I reached for my wallet to pay for my squash—and my chocolate biscotti—I began worrying whether I'd have time to go for a run.

The editors of checkout-counter magazines have a preternatural understanding of our inner battles over desire and self-restraint. They sell their product by allying themselves with both our cravings and our will to resist them. Like global arms merchants, they profit from the struggle. But some in medicine promise to free us from it. Obesity is an illness, they assure us— "a chronic, relapsing neurochemical disease," best managed with "automatic strategies" like drugs rather than "willpower" or "lifestyle changes."[7] To support their "disease" thesis, they point to chemical pathways—feedback loops from overstuffed fat cells to brain centers for appetite—gone awry. Fat is an endocrine tissue, researchers now know. It signals satiation by secreting a substance they've called leptin, and it shortens lives by releasing chemicals that raise blood pressure, worsen insulin resistance, and speed the build-up of arterial plaque.

I'm quite drawn to the prospect of reimagining corpulence as illness and dispensing with "willpower" as the treatment of choice. I'd love to avoid cardiac death, and I'd like brunettes in clingy jeans to crave me, without a long, twilight struggle against brownies and burgers. But, so far, I've held the waistline only with effort. No promising pill has come along. Appetite-suppressing stimulants have proven ineffective and dangerous. We know what works, when people can muster it: discipline and self-denial. Tight jeans may help too: Designer Karl Lagerfeld famously posed in a pair, for the cover of a diet book, to make the point that sexiness, explored through fashion, is a more pleasant motivator than fear. But as Lagerfeld, who lost 100 pounds, surely understood, saying no to tempting fare and pushing ourselves at the gym or on the jogging path are key.

So there's a case on health grounds against treating obesity as a disease, insofar as doing so discourages people from taking responsibility for calories consumed. But backers of the obesity-as-illness thesis tell powerful stories about both the biology of overeating and its social determinants. Plainly, the food industry, sedentary living, and the other usual suspects play causal roles.[8] And plainly, the incidence of weight problems has soared since the 1980s. About two thirds of Americans are overweight, and nearly a third are obese, as doctors have defined these terms.[9]

Supporters of the disease approach see these worrisome figures as reason for urgent action. Disease status, they say, will drive doctors and drug companies to develop new treatments, better than "willpower," by making health insurance available to cover them. More than that, it will encourage courts and legislators to use law as a public health tool against fast-food chains, the entertainment industry, and other enablers of our indulgence. Conservatives with a libertarian bent find these prospects appalling.[10] "Willpower," they hold, is a virtue in itself, not to be supplanted by neurochemicals. And lawsuits for "supersizing," or limits on fast-food advertising, represent nanny-state intrusion into people's lives.

Medical science can't resolve conflict over whether obesity is an illness. Claims to the contrary[11] mask the role of morals and politics in determining whether a condition counts as a disease. And in the case of obesity, money shapes the politics. Stomach-stapling surgeons and purveyors of diet pills want health plans to recognize obesity as an illness (and, of course, to pay for therapies); plans and employers have been understandably resistant. So has the food industry, worried that the disease model will unleash government's regulatory power. When in 2004, the federal agency that runs Medicare deleted a provision in its coverage manual stating that "obesity is not an illness,"[12] the head of an industry-backed advocacy group reproached the agency for "dumbing down" the idea of disease. "This is the only disease that I'm familiar with that you can solve by regularly taking long walks and keeping your mouth shut," he complained.[13] Meanwhile, a trade group representing sellers of obesity treatments boasted that its lobbying efforts played a critical role in convincing Medicare to change its policy.[14]

Medicine gives answers to the question of whether obesity and other conditions constitute illnesses by tapping political and cultural norms. In diagnosing and prescribing, doctors act as agents of norms that prevail.

Sometimes self-consciously, more often unwittingly, they both draw upon and shape popular understandings of what we should expect from society and what we owe ourselves. But the Hippocratic Myth doesn't permit doctors to acknowledge this. It commands them to act only on behalf of their patients—and, in so doing, puts their role as agents of society's norms ethically beyond the pale.

Do I Have a Right to Eat Brie?

The politics of personal responsibility also tacitly shapes treatment decisions and often underlies therapeutic controversies. Do I have a "right" to eat brie, boost my blood levels of artery-clogging LDLs (low-density lipoproteins, colloquially known as "bad cholesterol"), and then bother my doctor, at my employer's expense, for pricey medicine to bring my LDL levels down? Or should I first have to show restraint, holding off on the brie and buttery cookies (and doing hard time at the gym), before I'm able to tap my health insurance for thousands of dollars a year to pay for a prescription to lower my LDLs?

Different doctors answer this question in different ways, depending on the duties they think we owe ourselves. In seminars, conferences, and blogs, they argue over benefits and risks—over fragmentary data suggesting that LDL-lowering "statins" slow the growth of atherosclerotic plaque, make plaque less likely to kill by rupturing, and pose risks to liver, muscle, and memory. But underlying these arguments are more visceral disagreements, over our obligations to ourselves and our children, and over the good and bad that drug companies do.

Some doctors push statins as the first miracle drugs of the twenty-first century, an accomplishment as transformative as the antibiotic revolution sixty years earlier, and one for which drug firms deserve their rewards. (My own doctor says statins should be in the water supply.) Others offer a harsher take on human frailty and corporate greed. Opined one medical blogger: "We have a nation of overweight parents, addicted to processed foods and convenience foods, who are poisoning themselves and creating a nation of overweight, diabetic and cancer-prone children, and the answer of the American Academy of Pediatrics and the American Heart Association is to recommend a more aggressive use of cholesterol-lowering drugs."[15] Criticizing an article urging the benefits of statins even for people with normal cholesterol, another warned that "big pharma is behind the push to get as many people on statins as possible."[16]

Much more can and should be done to shield treatment decisions from drug company marketing muscle. But therapeutic judgment will always incorporate doctors' beliefs and biases about the promise of technology, the behavior and motives of commercial actors, and people's responsibilities to themselves. Our doctors are agents of these beliefs and biases, notwithstanding the Hippocratic Myth.

Consider, also, a scientific achievement that could save thousands of lives per year by preventing asthma attacks. In 2003, the FDA approved the sale of omalizumab, a genetically engineered protein with an unpronounceable name and a miraculous quality: It attaches to the chemical in our immune system that triggers asthma attacks. Once it does so, omalizumab acts like a safety catch, preventing this chemical, Immunoglobulin E, from setting off attacks.[17] Treatment would save most of the five thousand or so Americans who die from their asthma each year—if they could afford it. That's the rub: omalizumab, sold as Xolair by the drug firm Novartis, is extremely expensive—$5,000 to $10,000 a year for a minimal dose and up to $30,000 per year for larger doses.

By contrast, conventional therapy for persistent asthma is cheap—at most, several hundred dollars a year. And for most asthma sufferers, it's remarkably effective. But it won't "rescue" patients from attacks in progress[18]; it acts by preventing them. The mainstay of conventional treatment is an inhaled steroid[19] (there are several choices) that works by suppressing allergic reactions in the lungs—if it's used for weeks or months on end, whenever patients are at risk for attacks. This is a hassle for patients. They have to remember to use their inhalers a few times a day, whether they're wheezing or not. Many forget. Others don't bother, especially if days or weeks have passed since their last attack. Only about a quarter of Americans with asthma who should be on inhaled steroids (according to widely endorsed practice protocols[20]) actually use them.[21] Some can't afford them. Others aren't offered them.[22] Many more, though, are, in the argot of doctors, non-compliant.

Omalizumab offers a solution. It's given once a month, by injection, eliminating the need to remember or to bother. It would surely save lives, perhaps thousands of them, by preventing attacks in people who forget to inhale. That's cause for giving omalizumab to the non-compliant, some doctors say, and reason for health insurers to cover it as "medically necessary." But others insist that non-compliance not be rewarded with access to tens of thousands of dollars a year from our pooled health insurance premiums. Omalizumab, they argue, is a last-ditch drug for patients whom standard treatment fails. And treatment failure, they say, shouldn't be stretched to encompass self-neglect.

Different understandings of personal responsibility obviously drive this disagreement over clinical need. One can tell forgiving, causal stories about why people facing life's daily pressures forget or don't bother to take their steroids. Or one can insist that, irrespective of causal mechanisms, adherence to treatment that's cheap, low-risk, and life-saving is an obligation physicians and health plans should enforce by refusing to prescribe and pay for alternatives that cost much more. Either way, "medical necessity" here is a matter of morals and politics—politics doctors impose through their clinical decisions.

The Other R-word

The politics that underlie medical judgment turn quite nasty at times, no more so than when race is involved. I had the privilege to serve, some years back, on an Institute of Medicine committee on racial and ethnic disparities in health care. These disparities are large, even after researchers adjust for the most important cause—the fact that blacks, Latinos, and other disadvantaged groups are disproportionately represented among America's 50 million uninsured. Blacks with coverage get worse care than whites for cardiovascular disease, diabetes, many cancers, and other illnesses. We assembled a vast body of literature to document these disparities, then we sought to explain them.[23] In so doing, we angered many, from across the ideological spectrum. Some took offense at our failure to name and blame racism: Raw bigotry explained the differences, they said, and we'd covered it up by not uttering the word. Others blamed us for being divisive by speaking of "bias" and thus hinting at racism.

We did indeed speak of bias—of impressions that clinicians form subconsciously, based on cues that include race. We alluded to abundant evidence that conscious, reasoned decision making plays only a small part in people's judgment and that we rely, for the most part, on mental shortcuts, known as heuristics, to navigate life's complexity. Heuristics are often unconscious, and they're remarkably useful. They bridge the gap between our limited cognitive capacity and the sea of information that's around us.[24] We can't walk or drive, let alone cross busy intersections, without relying on uncountable prejudgments about the movement of people and vehicles. There are places we look and possibilities we disregard as we move forward, managing the risks. The complexity of human physiology gives heuristics an outsize role in medical practice.[25] But when race and ethnicity come into play as triggers for heuristics, prejudgments become prejudices, and matters become dicey.

The other "R-word," racism, misses the nuance. Sure, there are old-fashioned bigots—Jim Crow throwbacks who think blacks, Latinos, or whoever are less worthy. And there are disparities in empathy, irrespective of conscious intent—disparities that disfavor members of groups least represented among health professionals. My white, Yale-trained internist, who loves talking about health policy and prefers Democrats, probably finds it easier to connect with me than with someone who must make do, every day, amid the violence and poverty of the South Bronx streets. Empathy matters not only because we want our doctors to care; it steers scarce clinical resources toward those whom doctors care most about.

More pervasive prejudgments, though, arise from race-related preconceptions about patients' preferences, needs, and social situations. For example, it's folk wisdom among many physicians that African Americans are more skeptical than whites toward high-tech treatments and thus less likely to comply. And there's a widespread impression, not without some truth, that blacks are less likely to have the family support needed to endure aggressive treatments. (Thus, for instance, African American men are less likely to receive bypass surgery for blocked coronary arteries.) Doctors act on these preconceptions, incorporating them into decisions about whether to recommend more or less onerous measures, or any treatment at all.

In so doing, they make tacit distributive judgments—judgments that allocate diminished resources to disadvantaged minority groups. Rather than pushing beyond race-based preconceptions by putting more effort into learning about each patient, they rarely entertain doubts. And rather than allocating resources to offset disadvantage—by, say, providing extra home care services to patients with weaker family support—the health care system compounds social disadvantage by withholding some state-of-the-art therapies because of it.

To the extent that African Americans are less inclined to trust high-tech treatments (and doctors and hospitals in general), it's reasonable to ask why. There's abundant evidence that this "preference" for less vigorous treatment is a product of our country's tragic racial history. From 1932 until 1972, a quarter-century after antibiotics became widespread, U.S. Public Health Service researchers pressed ahead with an infamous study of the long-term effects of untreated syphilis in several hundred black men. Many died; others suffered catastrophic deterioration of brain function. Still others infected their wives or lovers. Had a whistleblower not tipped off the national media in 1972, the study might have gone on longer. For white Americans, "the legacy of Tuskegee," as the scandal's fallout came to be called, was a regulatory regime aimed at protecting human subjects of research, mainly by requiring their informed consent. But for African Americans, the legacy was lasting distrust of doctors and the health care system.[26]

Insensitive, hard-to-navigate hospital bureaucracies have deepened this distrust, as has the chasm between the social backgrounds of most physicians and many of the black people they serve. The alchemy of patience, warmth, politeness, and, when necessary, ability to make unhelpful bureaucrats sweat eludes many of us when we're dealing with miscreant mail-order clerks or cable companies. It's much harder when you fear for your life, you can't get through to the clinic, and the operator keeps transferring you to a non-working number. And it's even more difficult, and more intimidating, when the people with whom you're dealing are in castes above you and go by routines and rituals alien to those you know.

When it emerged during the 2008 presidential primary that Barack Obama's one-time pastor, the Reverend Jeremiah Wright, said doctors "invent[ed] the HIV virus as a means of genocide against people of color,"[27] most denounced Wright for spreading a canard that imperils African Americans' health by discouraging them from seeking care. But Wright was merely channeling a widespread impression. Polls have shown that double-digit percentages of blacks believe this[28]—a measure of the distrust many feel toward their doctors and hospitals.

That distrust, and the trials and humiliations many experience when making their way through our health system, depresses the level and quality of the care that African Americans receive. The Institute of Medicine committee on which I served saw this as a deep injustice—an inheritance from our nation's history of race-based contempt and disregard, even if not the product of current bigotry. But some say this view is paternalistic, even offensive, because it refuses to defer to African Americans' "preferences" for less intensive care. More than that, it's been urged that African Americans and others who don't seek the best, life-prolonging care for themselves and their loved ones act irresponsibly and have themselves to blame.

A common theme in these conservative critiques is that people make health care choices that doctors should honor. The reasons for these choices, the critics say, are beside the point. Clark Havighurst, a retired law professor at Duke who was once Ronald Reagan's health policy advisor,[29] complained to me that the Institute of Medicine panel missed the real unfairness: blacks who prefer less care pay the same insurance premiums as whites and thus subsidize whites' higher use of health services. The remedy, he told me, is cheaper health plans for those who want less care.

Whether clinical judgment should incorporate these purported African-American "preferences" for less care or aspire toward therapeutic equity is a political question. It's my belief that we owe black Americans—and members of other disadvantaged groups—an effort to address the fear and distrust that have led so many to miss out on life-extending care and clinical relationships. The best health systems are patient friendly. They're proactive about encouraging patients to come for preventive care. And they ensure that a doctor takes charge of coordinating care and otherwise helping people to find their way through bureaucratic thickets.[30]

So I reject the view that avoidance, motivated by fear and distrust, should be taken as a "preference" rather than treated as a moral challenge.[31] But either way, what's inescapable is that medical judgment incorporates doctors' beliefs about patient responsibility and social injustice. In assimilating these beliefs, doctors act as agents of contending political and moral visions, contrary to Hippocratic ideals. Since they're doing something they're not supposed to, they're loath to talk about it. And we're left with heated arguments that shed no light, about whether doctors are racist or just practicing good medicine by meeting their patients' varied needs.

Jeans Cruz

Heated arguments over the moral content of clinical judgment do sometimes effect change. Outrage over army doctors' use of personality disorder diagnoses to muster out Jeans Cruz and others with stress symptoms forced the Pentagon to change course on provision of medical and disability benefits to veterans with these symptoms. The Pentagon neither revised its diagnostic criteria for PTSD nor acknowledged the role of competing beliefs about martial courage, character, or who should bear the cost of combat. Both the Defense Department and its critics in Congress maintained the fiction that proper diagnosis of PTSD is a purely scientific matter, divorced from politics. So did the Institute of Medicine, when it rebuffed the Bush administraton's effort to raise the bar for the diagnosis. Yet army psychiatrists clearly changed direction, as did their VA colleagues. Without saying so, they began to decide the underlying moral questions differently, finding space to do so within the APA diagnostic manual's ambiguities.

This shift enabled Jeans Cruz to gain the medical benefits he badly needed. But that's not been enough for a storybook ending. Through 2008, his health steadily declined. Worsening asthma, loss of bladder control, and blood in his urine confounded his doctors—when he could make it in to the Bronx VA see them. It's just four miles from his home to the VA—a ten-minute drive but a day-long expedition for someone wheelchair-bound and reliant on public transit. Back spasms and severe pain punctuated his days. Terrifying memories continued to pursue him when he slept. Cruz's doctors pushed changing cocktails of drugs that seemed to do nothing. His bitterness deepened. His hopes as a father, a husband, and a provider for his family ebbed.

In Iraq's Sunni Triangle, where he'd stalked Saddam, passions cooled and quiet set in. But on the streets of the South Bronx, downstairs from his apartment, the war went on, among drug dealers vying for turf and gang members who'd given up on the future. Bullets flew and men died, blurring the distinction between traumatic memory and mayhem in real-time. Cruz lost contact with army buddies, congressional aides, veterans' activists, and others who'd helped him to beat Dr. Gray's personality disorder diagnosis. By the summer of 2009, getting out of bed had become a struggle. Keeping his doctors' appointments had become an iffy proposition. His phone number, which he'd given me on a business card with a billowing flag and the words "brothers in arms," had been disconnected, then assigned to someone else.

"It's an emotional battle that I feel like I'm losing," he'd told me the previous April. When I e-mailed him at the end of July to see how he was doing, he replied: "i have been extreamly ill lately i am on best rest most of the time i am getting better, but not so fast [*sic*]." He offered to call me for a brief chat, but he didn't follow up. He'd wanted me to talk with his doctors—to find out what they knew and might be able to do about his mystifying ailments. But he never did the necessary paperwork, paperwork that's meant to protect privacy but that's daunting even for the highest-functioning among us. He'd also wanted me to find him a lawyer, someone to take his case *pro bono* and set his military records right. But he became increasingly difficult to contact, inaccessible, as a practical matter, for all but the most persistent. The man whom family members had called a "ghost" was again disappearing, into a private universe of anger and despair.

chapter six

setting limits by consent

Mrs. Pearson

Mrs. Pearson's quiet self-possession, as she asked me to allow her to die, is what I most remember about her.[1] She was a trim African-American woman in her late fifties, elegant even in her wrinkled hospital gown. Her wavy gray hair had a just-shampooed luster, and she spoke with serenity, enunciating each syllable slowly, softly, but fully. I'd been called to her bedside because her doctor wanted a note in the chart from a psychiatrist, saying she was competent to stop dialysis. Doing so would mean death within a few weeks. She'd poison herself with her own blood—with the waste materials she couldn't clear, since her kidneys had shut down.

My first ten minutes with Mrs. Pearson convinced me that there was no question of her competence. She talked sensibly about the pain, inconveniences, and utter boredom she'd endured for years on dialysis. She organized most of her days around the hours she spent sitting beside a mechanical kidney, fat needles inside her, needles that took her blood to and from her body through ugly, always-open wounds. She dreaded each session for hours in advance; then there was the pain afterward from her fresh wounds. Quite simply, she said, it had become too much.

Mrs. Pearson wasn't merely rational; she was eloquent about the balance of burdens and benefits, as she saw it. She'd given it all a great deal of thought—more so than many of us give even our most momentous life choices, about whom to marry, what career path to take, or how to die. She didn't seem depressed; nor did she show what psychiatrists call "vegetative signs" of depression—trouble falling asleep, early-morning awakening, and loss of appetite. She'd contemplated her life circumstances free from the distorting effects of despairing sentiment. What she saw was too much suffering, stretching out too far into the future, for too little purpose.

I went through the motions of my mental status exam: "What's today's date? Where are we right now? Who's the president?"—that sort of thing. I did the rudimentary tests of abstract thinking, asking the meaning of hackneyed expressions like "people who live in glass houses shouldn't throw stones." I needed answers for the chart. She gave all the right ones, readily.

From an ethical point of view, my duty was clear. If Mrs. Pearson grasped the stakes, and was alert and oriented, she had a right to refuse treatment. She passed these tests easily. The dialysis would have to stop. It was my job to write the note saying so. Without a competent patient's informed consent, no test or treatment is ethical—at least none more intrusive than a needle stick or a Tylenol at bedtime. Mrs. Pearson was withdrawing her consent, and she was as mentally competent as I.

From Hippocratic Fidelity to Informed Consent

Informed consent is a recent creation. Until the 1970s, conventional wisdom among clinicians was that they needn't seek their patients' permission to act. Hippocratic benevolence, they held, was the best assurance that doctors would do right by their patients. And doing right didn't mean doing what patients said they wanted: Doctors often knew better. On behalf of their patients, doctors could coax and cajole by withholding some truths and inventing others. They could lie about bad prognoses and terrifying treatment risks. All this was justified by sick people's medical ignorance, childlike dependence, and disabling fears. And it was justified by doctors' intimate knowledge of their patients' hopes, worries, and quirks of character. The country doctor who rode circuit, visiting family farms, and the urban general practitioner who cared for mother and father and son and daughter over many years, developed rich understandings of their patients' lives. Or so the standard story held.

Informed consent originated as a way around the problem of breach of Hippocratic fidelity when physicians experiment on human beings. The Hippocratic tradition forbade such science. For centuries, settled wisdom held that a doctor could try a new treatment only to seek a better result for his patient. Doctors tried novel therapies based on hunch and hope. The scientific method requires more. It demands that recipients of a new treatment be compared with clinically similar controls—that is, with patients who are given conventional therapy, or no therapy at all. And ideally—to avoid the confounding influence of hope—it calls for keeping both doctors and patients in the dark about who is getting experimental therapy, conventional treatment, or neither. The scientific method thereby transforms patients from ends into means—means for accumulating knowledge about what will work best for others. It's thus at odds with the physician's Hippocratic pledge to her patients. It compromises their needs so that doctors can do better for other patients, down the line.[2]

So it's hardly surprising that physicians were slow to take up the scientific method. Not until the nineteenth century, in France, did medicine start down this path. A French physician, Pierre Louis, developed the first mathematical methods for comparing clinical results in experimental and control groups.[3] In 1835, he dismayed colleagues by publishing his finding that bloodletting failed to improve outcomes for patients with pneumonia. But neither Louis nor his contemporaries came up with an answer to the conflict between the research physician's Hippocratic and scientific roles. Some ignored this problem; others denied it, suggesting that human subjects of research weren't patients, especially when the research stood no chance of benefiting them.

Physician-researchers who admitted to their role conflict problem offered two ways out. The first—the heroic solution—called for doctors themselves to become human subjects. In 1900, U.S. Army Maj. Walter Reed led a research mission to Cuba to test the theory that biting mosquitoes spread yellow fever, which had killed thousands during the war with

Spain. The team allowed local mosquitoes to feed on yellow fever patients; then the researchers exposed themselves. The bugs bit again, and one of the doctors died. This, though, was hardly enough to prove that the insects were to blame. To establish that mosquitoes transmitted the disease, more human subjects were needed, many more than Dr. Reed's four-man team could provide.

So Reed's team turned to Cuban volunteers—and to the second of the two ways of coping with the conflict between their Hippocratic obligations and their research role. Reed and his colleagues asked each prospective volunteer to "endanger his life to a certain extent" by "tak[ing] the chance of contracting [yellow fever] intentionally." They offered, in exchange, "the greatest care and the most skill-ful medical service" plus "the sum of $100 in American gold"—and a second $100 for volunteers who came down with the disease.[4] Ethics scholars would later chide Reed for spinning his subjects by telling them they'd get yellow fever for sure if they didn't participate, since they lived on the island. But Reed's study, which proved that mosquitoes carry the disease,[5] marked the first formal, large-scale use of informed consent to manage conflict between research physicians' Hippocratic and scientific roles.

Over the next several decades, informed consent was rarely sought. Leading American physician-researchers opposed making it mandatory.[6] Through the 1930s, they fought off lawmakers' and professional societies' efforts to do so. It is, as bioethics scholar Albert Jonsen notes, the stuff of sour irony that Germany took the lead in requiring informed consent. A Prussian regulation passed in 1900 forbade non-therapeutic experimentation on human subjects without their consent "on the basis of a proper explanation of the adverse consequences that may result. . . ." More detailed rules requiring consent issued from the Reich Minister of the Interior in 1931, two years before Hitler took power.[7]

When, in 1947, the "Doctors' Trial" at Nuremberg concluded in verdicts against Karl Brandt and fifteen others for ghoulish experiments that have since defied understanding, the judges relied on wishful thinking, in the form of an AMA-appointed ethicist's claim that the rules governing research on human subjects were "well-established by custom, social usage, and the ethics of medical conduct." The judges embraced his account of these rules, announcing, in their opinion, that "[t]he voluntary consent of the human subject is absolutely essential."[8] But it wasn't "custom" for physician-researchers to require consent from their patients,[9] either for studies of new treatments or for participation in experiments that offered no therapeutic benefits.[10] Most clung to the belief that role conflict wasn't a problem. Hippocratic devotion to patients, backed by personal virtue, was all the protection their patients needed.[11]

So the judgment at Nuremberg that resulted in the hanging of seven Nazi physicians rested on a rule American doctors didn't apply to themselves. Through the 1940s and 1950s, American physicians injected plutonium into patients, exposed them to deadly infections, and challenged their bodies and minds with hormones and hallucinogens—all without their knowledge.[12] U.S. researchers all but ignored what came to be called the "Nuremberg Code"—rules endorsed by the "Doctors' Trial" judges as reason for condemning Brandt and his colleagues to die. The cornerstone of the Code, the "voluntary consent of the human subject," was an expedient for "barbarians," not medical men of good character.[13] "Nazis" weren't ethically relevant to "us."

That the 1950s were a highpoint for public trust in medicine—and in American institutions more generally—encouraged this complacency. But the 1960s brought disorienting change. Scandal played a large role, against a backdrop of rising civil rights consciousness and skepticism toward authority.[14] In 1966, a Harvard anesthesiologist aroused his colleagues' anger and many patients' worst fears with an article in the *New England Journal of Medicine* reviewing twenty two published instances of research he found unethical. Some were horror stories, involving intentional exposure of patients to danger, withholding of effective treatment, and exploitation of the poor and mentally disabled. Amidst rising public pressure to act, research leaders rediscovered the Nuremberg Code. Public officials weighed regulatory options. The character and conscience of the individual doctor would no longer do.

Following the logic of the Nuremberg Code, researchers and regulators seized upon informed consent as the solution. But this was more a finesse than an answer to the core problem—the research physician's rival commitments as caregiver and scientist. Rather than confronting the role conflict problem head-on, the informed-consent response reframed it as a matter of safeguarding personal choice. Research doctors had double agendas, the thinking went, but patients, acting freely, could protect themselves. This solution fit the ethos of the 1960s: Personal autonomy would be the antidote for authoritarian overreach.

Left behind was another approach—one that would have eliminated the role conflict altogether. In 1951, Dr. Otto Guttentag, a German physician who'd fled to American just months after the Nazis took power, proposed that the role of research physician be split up, into "physician-experimenter" and "physician-friend." "[R]esearch and care should not be pursued by the same person," he argued. The experimenter's purpose is "not to help but to confirm or disprove. . . ." The caregiver's responsibility is to stand in "solidarity" with his patient.[15]

Guttentag's idea gained a hearing but no traction. It would have been costly—an additional doctor (the "friend") would have had to be hired for each patient. More than that, it would have been contentious. It would have brought the role conflict into the open, in the form of adversary relations between experimenter and "friend." Research physicians would have had to endure constant, close oversight from sophisticated colleagues. The informed-consent solution, by contrast, kept the role conflict under wraps, constraining physicians only to the extent that their patient-subjects said "no." And patients asked to consent, it would turn out, were quite pliable.

Beyond that, the "physician-friend" had been left behind in another sense. As medicine advanced from the days of home visits, made on horseback, to high technology, delivered in hospitals, doctors became strangers to their patients, especially at moments of dire need. I've counted at least four books, by distinguished scholars of medical ethics and law, with "Strangers" in their titles.[16] All play on the paradox of intimate relations between the sick and specialists unfamiliar with their patients' lives, loves, and fears. Doctors who encounter sick people as strangers and focus on single physiological systems make for unlikely "physician-friends." Informed consent was a better match for medicine's new technocratic mindset. Doctors who maintained only minimal, transient relationships with their patients could reveal risks and request consent.

Over the course of a decade, from the mid-sixties through the mid-seventies, informed consent to clinical research became standard practice, mandated by a catalog of federal regulations. Each fresh scandal, it seemed, set off a new cycle of inquiries, legislation, and rulemaking. Ethicists and legal scholars, meanwhile, built a conceptual framework for the governance of research that put personal autonomy at the center.[17] Federal regulators embraced this framework,[18] which relied upon the abstractions of analytic philosophy rather than the Hippocratic promise of loyalty and care. Compassion at the bedside became "beneficence." Doctors' discredited claims of virtue were supplanted by the Kantian ideal of "respect for persons," which meant, in practice, protection for autonomy. And the intricate reasoning of philosophers sat well with a new generation of physician-researchers who saw themselves as technocrats, had high regard for expertise, and were inclined to treat ethics as another subspecialty. Medical schools created departments of bioethics and staffed them with scholars trained in philosophy and law. The nuanced analyses these scholars produced shaped regulatory policy and research design.

In the 1970s, informed consent made a further leap, from clinical research to medical care more generally. Judges insisted upon it, and a new generation of doctors embraced it.[19] They'd learned in medical school to talk to their patients about risks and benefits and to allow them to say no. My visit to Mrs. Pearson's bedside was occasioned by her doctors' assumption that she could say no to further dialysis, so long as she grasped the consequences.

A Hard Right Turn

Political liberals were at the forefront of the informed consent revolution. They drew energy and inspiration from campaigns for personal freedom in realms from civil rights to sexual fulfillment. But in the 1980s, informed consent took a hard right turn. Free-market conservatives invoked it as the solution to a problem that business and government had begun to notice but that bioethics had ignored—the rise of health spending.

Already by the late seventies, there was much talk of a medical cost "crisis." Health insurers were under pressure to stop writing blank checks to doctors and hospitals, then billing employers. And for the first time, they began to say no. Some added small print to their contracts, empowering them not to cover care prescribed by patients' physicians. Others went further, insisting that doctors get their permission before performing tests and treatments. These steps were unheard of in the sixties and seventies: Insurers simply paid for whatever the treating physician said was needed.[20] But by the early 1980s, insurer involvement of this sort had become commonplace. Physicians resented this new affront. Insurers, they warned, were interfering with their Hippocratic duty to do the best they could for their patients. Patients, in turn, worried about having to choose between the risks of forgoing treatment and being stuck with huge bills.

Market-oriented commentators offered an intrepid response. Rather than standing in the way of doctors' Hippocratic obligations, they said, insurers' assertiveness helped to fulfill them, by keeping doctors from spending too much. The new policies enabled patients to choose in advance to economize on care, by signing insurance contracts that authorized health plans to set limits. Only by setting such limits could insurers hold prices down. And by accepting these limits, physicians honored their Hippocratic pledge, since patients *chose* these limits when they signed up for coverage.

The key move here, as Clark Havighurst (who pioneered this rationale) pointed out, was to shift the locus of consent from the bedside to the moment when people sign up for health plans. It's right to do so, Havighurst said, because people take account of costs as well as benefits when they buy coverage. In the hospital, by contrast, they're playing with the house's money (once they reach their maximum copayments and deductibles), so they have no incentive to weigh costs. They have every reason to seek all care that might be of benefit, so long as they can stick their insurers with the bill. So honoring (and enforcing) the choices people make when signing up respects their freedom to choose how to spend their money.[21]

Thus physicians face no role conflict, by this line of reasoning, when they set limits on health plans' behalf. By so doing, doctors honor their patients' preferences. Enforcing limits on coverage affirms patients' freedom to bind themselves. Without such enforcement, insurance couldn't work as a business proposition, since insurers would have to write checks for care they didn't count on covering.

In the 1980s and 1990s, health plans became more aggressive. They paid doctors to withhold care and refused to cover pricey treatments. The cost-saving stratagems I discussed in chapters two and three became routine. In courtrooms, congressional hearings, and other arenas, health plans and their hired advocates continued to press the claim that they were keeping faith with patients by honoring their contractual commitments.

But there was a chasm between this consent-in-theory and actual practice. Health plans revealed next to nothing about their cost-control policies. Most fought to keep their criteria for paying claims *secret,* saying they didn't want doctors and patients to be able to "game the system." Most said nothing to subscribers—not even in the small print—about their rewards to physicians for withholding care. Behind the veil of "medical necessity" clauses in their contracts with patients, they exercised vast discretion to say no.

A few free-marketeers chided health plans for failing to give meaning to "medical necessity" by clarifying the cost-benefit trade-offs they made. But most didn't fret about the disconnect between the industry's close-to-the-vest approach to cost control and the disclosure needed to claim that patients consented to rationing policies when they signed up for coverage. *Informed* consent to limit-setting practices wasn't being sought or obtained. Insurers weren't telling potential customers that they rationed care or enticed doctors to do so. So they had no plausible basis for claiming that patients consented by contract to their limit-setting policies and methods.

To the insurance industry's dismay, courts called it to account for this. Some judges rejected insurers' assertions that "medical necessity" clauses in their contracts allowed doctors to weigh costs. Courts were similarly hostile when health plans kept mum about enticements to skimp on care. In one high-profile case, forty-year-old Patrick Shea implored his family-practice doctors over an eight-month period to refer him to a cardiologist for chest pain, dizziness, and shortness of breath. The doctors, Sidney Esensten and Jeffrey Arenson, told him it wasn't necessary. They ascribed his symptoms variously to anxiety and stomach problems. On March 5, 1993, Shea phoned his wife Dianne, told her he again felt chest pain, then drove to see his doctors. He was found dead, slumped over the steering wheel, several blocks from their clinic.

An autopsy revealed severe coronary disease, almost certainly the cause of death. And an inquiry by the lawyers Dianne retained discovered that the Sheas' health plan paid bonuses to Esensten and Arenson for limiting referrals to specialists. Her lawyers asserted in federal court that the plan had a duty to disclose these enticements. A trial judge found otherwise, but the Eighth Circuit Court of Appeals reversed, ruling that the payments were "material" to her late husband's health concerns and should have been disclosed.[22] And when, three years later, the U.S. Supreme Court said in *Pegram v. Herdrich* that an HMO's rewards to doctors for withholding care were a permissible "inducement to ration," the justices suggested (without reaching the issue) that the HMO had a duty to disclose them.

The Logic of Consent—and Its Limits

Were health plans to reveal their rationing policies to potential customers, would consent before-the-fact, through the decision to subscribe, justify doctors' commitment to these policies even when their patients protest? Put differently, does consumer choice at the point of sign-up deserve a privileged position over patient preference once illness arises? And is it plausible to say that doctors, in such circumstances, fulfill their Hippocratic obligation by keeping faith with the former at the expense of the latter?

These are values questions, not answerable through logical syllogism. Common sense, though, commands acknowledgment that limit setting is essential and that uncompromising commitment to the sick patient's perspective renders it impossible. Insurance is a wrinkle not envisioned by the writers of the Oath—or by the physicians who swore fealty to it in centuries past. Keeping faith with patients who pay their own way calls for sensitivity to their financial circumstances—to the balances they strike between medical care and other needs. So, absent insurance, the Oath requires that doctors take account of costs. Add insurance to the mix, though, and the patient's costs disappear from the calculus of Hippocratic duty, since someone else is footing the bill. Unless, that is, we reinterpret the Oath as a commitment to the perspective of the patient when she signed up for coverage and (presumably) paid heed to insurance prices.[23]

Doing so hardly sweeps away the subjective sense of breach of faith, even abandonment, a patient may feel when a doctor withholds potentially lifesaving care because its costs don't comport with an insurer's trade-off policies. But if these policies are made vivid and clear to all who sign up for coverage, and if consumers have a decent menu of low- and high-cost coverage options (with differing cost-benefit trade-off rules), then this breach of faith is defensible.

These are, though, large "ifs." What does it take to make a health plan's cost-benefit balancing principles so vivid and clear to consumers when they sign up that we can say they've consciously chosen to abide by them? Should health plans be required by law to adopt a single, shared way of declaring their trade-off policies—say, maximum dollar amounts per expected life year that they'll spend on tests and treatments? How about a checklist of representative services, ranging from urgent-care services to screening tests, that are or aren't covered? And how much choice between health plans (and trade-off rules) is enough to make for a decent menu of options? Finally, what should be done about disparities in wealth? Is there a decent minimum of buying power (and public subsidies) below which real choice between trade-off rules isn't possible? These are matters of policy and politics, beyond my scope in this book. But they'll need to be become the focus of public attention, leading to agreement, if we're to enlist the nation's support for limit-setting by health plans and their doctors.

To some Hippocratic purists, any collusion by clinical caregivers with rationing policies is unacceptable.[24] The Oath, they insist, demands that doctors keep faith with sick patients, not with insurers' limit-setting rules. But even if we refuse to read the Oath as a commitment to rationing policies previously agreed to by the sick, requiring doctors to comply with these policies is justifiable. Professional loyalty plays out within bounds—within rules set by social institutions that accommodate competing claims. Within hospitals, physician-administrators decide who gets priority for intensive care beds and other scarce resources. A clinical caregiver can make the case for her patients, but she cannot lie about lab results; nor can she simply impose her will, say, by wheeling a patient into the cardiac care unit over the unit chief's objections. Likewise, lawyers have an ethical duty to press their clients' cases with zeal, but this doesn't entitle them to present forged documents or false testimony. Lawyers are "officers of the court," subject to court rules. Clinical limits set in legitimate fashion, whether by patient consent before the fact or other means, define the boundaries of Hippocratic obligation, just as the rules of evidence and procedure specify the outer limits of lawyerly advocacy.

Rewards to doctors for stinting on care are another matter. There's a clear difference between setting outer bounds on what doctors can do for their patients and enticing physicians to break faith. The doctor who tells her patient that she's tried but failed to win coverage for breast MRI or endometriosis surgery delivers disappointing news. But the physician who takes money for *not* pursuing pricey options leaves her patients with the bitter taste of betrayal—if they find out. The former sort of disappointment is inherent in the task of setting limits. Betrayal, though, is unnecessary, and it's toxic to the doctor-patient relationship.

This isn't to say that frugality shouldn't count. Payment schemes that encourage sensible, science-based care—care premised on the cost-benefit balances people strike when they buy coverage—can nudge doctors toward parsimony without suborning them to break faith. There's a critical difference between performance standards tied to trade-offs accepted by plan members and rewards to doctors for withholding care regardless of health consequences. The former encourage doctors to stick to the deal their patients struck. The latter incite disloyalty and arouse public ire.

How far the logic of consent can be carried to sanction saying no on account of cost is a matter of practical judgment, not pure reason. My conclusion that before-the-fact consent to rationing principles can justify doctors' adherence to them reflects both my alarm about soaring medical costs and my confidence that asking physicians to follow rules won't leave patients feeling betrayed. And my judgment that monetary enticements to doctors for withholding care go too far rests on my sense that *motives* matter: Patients will more readily accept bad news about limits from physicians who champion their needs, albeit within the rules, than from doctors motivated by money to skimp.

That the logic of consent has its limits is something Mrs. Pearson taught me, unforgettably. After I finished going through the motions of my mental status exam, I went to the nurses' station to put a note in her chart, allowing her to die. I'm embarrassed to admit that I felt a sort of pride. I was about to put ethics into action—to walk the walk—to stand up, when it mattered, for patient self-determination. I'd document Mrs. Pearson's equanimity, her highly rational state of mind, and the conscientiousness she'd shown as she parsed the costs and benefits of continuing on dialysis.

There was no question of her competence to withdraw her consent. She was astonishingly rational, it seemed. Too rational? I stopped writing and went back to her room. She greeted me pleasantly. I asked her a few questions about her daughters, both in their twenties and, she reassured me, doing well. There were no family ruptures or rending disappointments. I then told her I wondered how her daughters might feel about losing her. Did they know, I asked, that their mom was about to die? She looked at me serenely, too serenely, and said they'd be sad but they'd deal with it. They didn't know yet, but they'd understand.

Did she want to leave them? I then asked. I knew I'd taken a risk. Was I offering Mrs. Pearson a vent for suppressed feeling, or was I just being provocative? I wasn't sure. No, she answered. She didn't want to. Her cheeks seemed to tighten; her voice did as well. Her serenity seemed to dissolve into quiet anger. They'll have to handle it, she said. She had to handle it, and she couldn't. Not the way the people who ran the dialysis unit expected her to. They'd just changed her schedule, she told me—without telling her in advance, without asking her what would and wouldn't work for her. No more night sessions. Something about it being too expensive. She'd have to come in more often, for shorter times. There'd be more pain—the hurt she felt each time the dialysis tech pushed the two fat needles into her forearm, sometimes moving them around to reach her squiggly, scarred veins.

The shift from night to day meant dialysis would become her main life project. That's, at least, how she experienced the rescheduling. Night sessions were a postscript to the day's events; day treatment would *be* the main event. Dialysis, some patients say, feels like a steamroller. And she'd have to face the steamroller, and the pain and dread beforehand, most days of the week. The hospital didn't care. The dialysis techs didn't care. And she had no say in the matter. Unless she said no to dialysis itself.

I figured, or hoped, that this was the point—gaining some say. I'd missed the point as I'd prepared to put ethics into action—to be a bioethics "hero" (in my imaginings) by writing a note affirming Mrs. Pearson's competence to bring her life to an end. So instead of going back to the nurses' station to finish my note, I asked her for permission to talk with the dialysis folks. She said sure, promising me I'd get nowhere.

I felt like a detective on a cold case as I tried to figure out who'd changed Mrs. Pearson's dialysis schedule and who might be able to switch it back. Nobody on the unit admitted to doing it. The doctors insisted they could do nothing—it was up to an administrator on a different floor, whom they didn't know. I forget how I finally found the culprit, a supervisor of some sort who'd gotten a talking-to about the hospital's annual deficit, the cost of the night sessions, and the need for everyone to endure a little inconvenience. I let him know the stakes in this case were higher. Mrs. Pearson had given me quite a trump card, and I played it as best I could. He'd been cutting back on the night hours, he told me. But there were some openings. He'd fit her in. And he'd let her keep the evening slots after she left the hospital.

I went downstairs to let her know. I fretted: Would my bit of political ward-healing be enough? Or would she come up with some other reason to say no, forcing me to follow the rules and confirm her competence to quit? What was really driving her? And was that any of my business? Wasn't it my duty to just do the bioethics "thing"—to write the note that'd empower her? Or was I doing right by trying to solve the mystery of her motives and to resolve matters that cookbook bioethics treated as beside the point?

I entered Mrs. Pearson's room, unable to hold back a grin. Like a ticket-fixing local pol, I'd delivered. I told her she was scheduled for dialysis the next evening, and for the evenings after that, for the fewer and longer sessions she'd previously undergone. I muttered something about bureaucrats, then said we'd need to let the dialysis folks know quickly if we wanted to keep the slots. She smiled, saying softly that she wanted to go ahead. The night sessions would work for her. They'd worked well enough in the past. She wasn't joyful or happy, but she did seem much-relieved. She offered a quiet thank-you, and I said goodbye. I told her I'd look for her, nights, on the dialysis unit, while I was still on the psych consult service.

I went to the nurses' station to find my partially written note. I put down my findings on the mental status exam, documented her competence to refuse dialysis, and said she'd decided to continue it for the foreseeable future. I checked back with the dialysis unit several days after, then weeks later. She was still showing up for her night sessions. I stopped by a few times, when I could grab a moment, but I never saw her again. That's part of the deal for doctor and patient at a vast academic medical center. We share life-and-death moments with each other, as strangers, then we part ways.

What happened to remix the options in Mrs. Pearson's mind, I don't know. But it surely had something to do with feeling acknowledged. I doubt the dialysis schedule in itself was a life-or-death matter. The hospital bureaucrats' utter disregard for her as an architect of her own life, though, surely was. Denied the chance for any say in the routine that both preserved and defined her daily existence, she asserted herself in the only way the system allowed. The law would have honored her decision to die. But it would have been wrong for me to take this choice at face value. It would have meant disregarding submerged states of mind—unrevealed feelings and beliefs—that might have nudged her decision in a different direction. And it would have meant accepting all the terms of the choice situation, including the administrators' imperious approach to her schedule.

The Preferences We Reveal

When it comes to our preferences, the law's gaze is skin deep: It registers only those that we reveal through our words and actions. Law honors the contracts we sign and the consent we make explicit—to doctors, lovers, and others. But below this level, people's desires and decisions are much messier. They're the product of states of mind—constellations of feeling and be-lief—that compete with each other to take command. Like political factions struggling for supremacy, these states of mind vie to shape the preferences we reveal to the law's gaze. Our decisions—the consent we give and the contracts we sign—are the outcomes of this rivalry within the mind. No ho-munculus—no single "self"—weighs factors and renders judgment. Indeed, a growing body of evidence from psychology and the neurosciences supports the conclusion that our sense of "self" is illusory.

More precisely, the "self" we experience is a composite—a fusion of sys-tems of cognition and emotion that both reinforce and compete with each other. Over the past quarter-century, cognitive psychologists have probed these systems with ingenious experiments. A common theme behind these experiments has been the manipulation of choice scenarios with an eye to-ward activating different mixes of reason and feeling. Change the mix, it turns out, and people choose differently, even though the options they're choosing between are *objectively* the same.

Consider an example that's become classic among cognitive psycholo-gists—the "Asian disease" scenario. Researchers tell volunteers to imagine that the government is preparing for the outbreak of an illness that's ex-pected to kill 600 people—if authorities do nothing. The volunteers are then split randomly into two groups. Volunteers in both groups are then asked to choose between two strategies, Program A and Program B, for reducing the toll. They're given precise information about each program's expected outcome—the number of lives each strategy would save. They're told nothing about how the programs actually would work. But—here's the key—the two groups are given different *descriptions* of the choice they're to make—that is, different explanations of each program's expected outcome.

The first group hears the following:

- If Program A is adopted, 200 people will be saved.
- If Program B is adopted, there is a one-third probability that 600 people will be saved and a two-thirds probability that no people will be saved.

The second group gets a different spin:

- If Program A is adopted, 400 people will die.
- If Program B is adopted, there is a one-third probability that nobody will die and a two-thirds probability that 600 people will die.

Again, the options are identical for each group: Program A reduces the disease's anticipated death toll from 600 to 400, while Program B has a one-third chance of saving all 600. (If this chance doesn't pan out, Program B saves nobody.) So we'd expect rational volunteers with stable "selves" to make the same choice, whichever version they hear. And we'd expect the two groups to prefer Program A and Program B by the same proportions, unaffected by how the options are spun.

But the spin matters greatly. The results differ dramatically. The first group chooses Program A by a large majority; the second group prefers Program B. Why? It's almost certainly because the stark depictions of Program A arouse passions not triggered by the probabilities of Program B. Saving 200 lives moves us more than Program B's uncertain payoff. Dooming 400 to die feels more tragic than giving each expected victim a fighting chance. These gut reactions activate neuronal networks—and states of mind—that drive decisions differently.

Evidence from brain-scanning studies demonstrates this. For the past decade or so, scientists have employed a technique known as functional magnetic resonance imaging (fMRI) to monitor activity levels in different brain areas while people make decisions. fMRI detects variations in blood flow to brain regions,[25] making it possible to track changes in neuronal activity, since neuronal firing increases blood flow. And it turns out that when experimental subjects are given problems like the Asian disease scenario, differences in "spin," or framing of the problem, tend to activate different brain regions. These different patterns of neuronal activation correlate with the choices that subjects make—choices that reflect different states of mind.

We're nowhere near to a thorough grasp of how these different states of mind shape a person's shifting sense of self. But we can confidently say that people make different choices, rooted in divergent understandings, when variations in the framing of a problem activate these different states. Deference to a person's announced choice begs the question of which framing of the problem should count. And as Mrs. Pearson's experience underscores, this can be a loaded question. The hospital's framing of her life-or-death decision (in particular, the hospital's imperious approach to her dialysis schedule) was morally unconscionable, in my view.

For Mrs. Pearson, the hospital's imperiousness was no less important than the schedule itself. It aroused her ire. It insulted her sense of dignity. That feelings of this sort can trump people's longer-standing goals and desires is illustrated by another psychologists' favorite: the "ultimatum game." I play it with my students by coming into class with a tasty surprise—irresistible to some (I confess it's irresistible to me): a thick bar of Swiss dark chocolate. I tear open the foil wrapping, then walk around the class with the chocolate, giving my students a chance to see, smell, and desire. I then ask who craves it maddeningly, choose the two who most persuade me, and bring both to the front of the room. They can share it, I tell them, if they play by my rules.

The bar, I point out, has six rows of chocolate, each divided into five squares. That's thirty in total, to be divided up—or forgone entirely—as follows: One of the two students takes temporary custody of the chocolate, but she must make an offer to the other. She can offer any number of squares she chooses, from zero to thirty. If her classmate accepts her offer, that's how the chocolate is divided: She gives him the squares she's offered and gets to eat the rest. But if the second student *declines* her offer, *I* take the chocolate bar back. Then I eat it—or if I'm afraid I'm gaining weight, I give it to the *rest* of the class to divvy up, while my two chocolate-craving volunteers endure the bitter without the sweet.

The most rational thing for the first student to do (to maximize her chocolate pleasure) is to offer a single square. Then she gets to eat the other twenty-nine, assuming her classmate accepts. And it's rational for him to do so; then he gets to eat a square of rich dark chocolate he'd otherwise go without. Surely (I chose him because he craves the stuff) he'd accept my *gift* of a single square if, instead of playing this peculiar game, I'd offered to break one off for him at the start. Yet students in the offeree's role almost always say no if asked to make do with just one square while their gluttonous classmate gets the other twenty-nine. They do so out of spite, since they're denying themselves the sweet dark moment they crave.

Perhaps, you might say, my students are particularly belligerent. They're law students, after all. But trials of the ultimatum game in diverse cultural settings yield consistent results. Offerees, as a rule, won't take less than 20 percent of the thing that's divvied up.[26] (In psychologists' experiments, it's typically money.) They'll go without, rather than be galled by getting less. We know it's about ire, not calculation, since in these experiments there aren't repeat plays. It might make sense, that is, to say no to a stingy offer so as to signal the offeror that she'd best be more generous next time. But if there's no next time—if offeror and offeree go their separate ways after a single round—then there's no point in saying no—no point, aside from spite.

Brain scanning studies confirm the triumph of spite over strategic thinking. Offerees monitored by fMRI as they reject low-ball offers show high activity in the anterior insula, a region linked in other studies to anger and disgust, and low activity in the dorsolateral prefrontal cortex, an area associated in prior research with sustained, goal-directed effort.[27] Feelings of unfairness about the options, it seems, throw our brains into altered states—states at war with more lasting commitments—to acquiring chocolate, accumulating money, or, in Mrs. Pearson's case, staying alive.

Had I accepted Mrs. Pearson's withdrawal of consent as her "choice," I'd have disregarded her unstated willingness to stay on dialysis, a willingness that persisted alongside her announcement to the contrary. That the law would have let me do so in the name of self-determination astonishes me. Doing so would have denied the import of the submerged beliefs, hopes, and commitments that inspired Mrs. Pearson, most days, to endure. There's a fuzzy line between rejecting old-style paternalism and ignoring the contradictions within ourselves—between our yearnings for respect, love, a sense of purpose, and life's other satisfactions. Treating people's on-the-spot decisions—in the marketplace and at the bedside—as proof of their enduring wants and needs disregards these contradictions and denies the context-dependence of people's choices.

Moreover, had I taken Mrs. Pearson's "choice" to die at face value, I'd have given the hospital a free pass to treat her in a fashion I thought unconscionable. To conclude that someone has chosen freely, we must make a prior judgment—moral or legal—about the sufficiency of her set of options. Consider philosophy's classic illustration of coercion—the highwayman who holds a traveler at gunpoint and offers a "choice": "Your money or your life." That's not a *real* choice, people say, because the options are coercive. But what makes them so? The would-be thief isn't physically overpowering his victim. He's not, somehow, seizing control of the traveler's arms like some wand-wielding foe of Harry Potter and forcing the arms (literally) to give over the wallet. He's offering the traveler two options: Hand over the money or die. (We're asked to assume that the traveler hasn't exercised her Second Amendment rights.)

We refuse to characterize the traveler's dilemma as a *choice* because the highwayman's threat is morally unacceptable. Consider, by contrast, a person just diagnosed with pancreatic cancer. She's told she must choose between certain death within a few months and extensive surgery that stands a decent chance of adding years to her life. She's under as much pressure to consent to the surgery as the traveler is to surrender his money; yet we don't treat her consent as coerced (bioethicists and courts, at least, don't). What's different? A bad diagnosis, not bad behavior, gave rise to the pressure. There's no culpable actor or wrongful action; her aggressive tumor is the product of cruel fate.

Likewise, the person who signs up for a health plan that sets limits *consents* to them, in the eyes of ethicists, if her range of insurance options is morally acceptable. If the choices her employer (or her country) gives her are insufficient, in our eyes, we say she's been coerced. Coercion, as the philosopher Alan Wertheimer points out, is a matter of moral baselines—baselines by which we assess the adequacy of the chooser's options.[28] So when we argue about whether someone has freely consented or has been coerced, we're really bickering over the baselines against which sets of options should be judged. If the hospital's cancellation of Mrs. Pearson's night dialysis sessions were a mere inconvenience—something she should have tolerated—then it's implausible to call her situation coercive. But if the schedule change was morally amiss, as I felt it was, her options fell below the baseline—not in a legal sense, but to my own way of thinking. That's what motivated me to try to remix her options. It wasn't just that canceling her night sessions made her life more trying. The administrator's way of doing so was an assault on Mrs. Pearson's sense of worth as a person.

If, though, the conclusion that a person has chosen freely is the byproduct of a prior judgment about the adequacy of her options, then consent does less work than it seems. As rationalization for role conflict, it's a shell game. Consent can't justify a doctor's double agenda as caregiver and arbiter of costs. Arguments over whether patients should be allowed to agree by contract to particular cost control measures reflect disagreements over the morality and necessity of these measures. Consent can neither dissolve nor finesse these differences.

Through politics and law—and, at times, public uproar—democratic societies must confront and accommodate these differences. Quiet deliberation among clinicians and ethicists won't suffice. The enormity of the stakes for all citizens will require much broader engagement if we're to reach accommodations that endure. Raucousness of the sort that makes policy wonks wince will be part of this process. The primal rants of talk show hosts, townhall participants, and myriad others are evidence of public engagement. So up to a point, dare I say, they're a good sign. But the crucial next step for political leaders is to rechannel this raucous engagement toward the large problems that democratic institutions have so far failed to manage. We'll need to go beyond the present paralysis on such contested questions as the care that ought to be available to all, the mix of public subsidies and private sacrifice necessary to pay for it, the right balance between benefits and costs, and how far we depart from Hippocratic ideals to achieve it. And to escape the current paralysis, we'll need to throw off the Hippocratic Myth, which has rendered pursuit of this balance unspeakable.

chapter seven

doctors as warriors I

america's frisson with torture

Dr. Uithol

On a chilly November night in 2003, a plane carrying army major Scott Uithol touched down in Baghdad after a steep, lights-out descent, meant to make a missile strike less likely. Uithol, a psychiatrist, was desperately needed. Armed resistance to America's presence was surging. Baghdad's streets had become deadly and terrifying. Battle stress symptoms were affecting a third or more of soldiers in many units, wearing away at their judgment and ability to fight. Dr. Uithol was set to deploy to a combat stress control team, tasked to treat soldiers traumatized by the terrors of urban warfare. But a day or so after landing in Baghdad, Uithol learned that his assignment had changed. On November 15, he reported to the Baghdad Central Confinement Facility, which would later become known to the world as Abu Ghraib.

For the next thirty-three days, Dr. Uithol served with the 205th Military Intelligence (MI) Brigade, advising interrogators intent on breaking their captives' will to resist. He was removed from his medical chain of command and assigned to lead Abu Ghraib's new "Biscuit," or behavioral science consultation team. What, precisely, he and the Biscuit did at Abu Ghraib remains a mystery—something he won't talk about, at least for the record, to this day. But Uithol's friends report that he went into a near panic over what MI expected him to do.

"When I got to Abu Ghraib," he told me years later, "I didn't know what a Biscuit was."[1] Close to clueless about interrogation, he tried an online search, seeking tips his clinical training hadn't provided. The MI chain of command wasn't much interested in what he found. Interrogation of "high-value" detainees by the men and women of the 205th didn't hew to traditional military or civilian approaches. The job of the Biscuit at Abu Ghraib was to craft and oversee schedules of sleeplessness, shackling, sexual insult, and other stressors to fit each uncooperative prisoner's personality and mood. That this role was at odds with doctors' duties as non-combatants under the Geneva Conventions seemed not to matter to the 205th's commander, Colonel Thomas Pappas. The Biscuit's mission was to develop personalized interrogation plans in collaboration with the 205th's Tiger teams—groups of interrogators assigned to high-value detainees. To put these plans into effect, interrogators instructed guards to strip and shackle prisoners, keep them awake according to prescribed schedules, and otherwise stress and debase them as directed.[2]

According to Pappas, Dr. Uithol wasn't a mere bystander. Pappas would later tell army investigators that interrogation plans "include a sleep plan and medical standards" and that "a physician and a psychiatrist are on hand to monitor what we are doing."[3] "As to what is implemented," Pappas claimed, the doctors "have the final say." To this end, said Pappas, Uithol would go to the cell blocks with interrogators, review detainees "under a management plan," and "provide feedback as to whether they were being medically and physically taken care of." Uithol's skills as a healer were thus pressed into service to support the combat mission—and to aid interrogation practices that flouted the laws of war.

The interrogation strategy he briefly oversaw was conceived long before he arrived at Abu Ghraib. Doctors designed it, administered it, and spread word about it to America's post-9/11 archipelago of interrogation sites. Doctors, moreover, were central to the Bush administration's efforts to legally justify it—and to protect its practitioners from criminal accountability for torture. Parts of this story are known from journalistic accounts and releases of once-secret materials. Other parts of the story are reported here for the first time, based on interviews with principals who haven't previously spoken, as well as documents newly obtained from participants and through the Freedom of Information Act.

Scott Uithol knew nothing of this history. "I'm excited about the mission," he told a colleague when he first learned of his surprise posting. Other army psychiatrists didn't share his enthusiasm. When word spread to the several other in-country psychiatrists that MI wanted one of them for Abu Ghraib, they pulled strings to avoid the assignment. Uithol welcomed it. "He's gung ho," another army colleague, also in Baghdad at the time, told me. "He bleeds army green. He's a decent guy who wants to do the right thing but sometimes gets a little overexcited."

Uithol's qualms came later, amid Abu Ghraib's chaos. Cut off from the army's medical chain of command, he had no senior colleagues to turn to as a counterweight to MI's expectations. And these expectations were without precedent in the history of American medicine. Saying "no" wasn't an option, as he saw things. He'd committed to the army as a career, and he wasn't about to wreck his prospects by disobeying an order or even intimating that he harbored doubts. But he read through the Geneva Conventions and decided that he shouldn't further confuse matters by providing medical care to detainees, as some at Abu Ghraib wanted him to do. "I'm not your doctor," he would tell prisoners he encountered. "I'm with the guys with the guns."

Later, Uithol would look back on Abu Ghraib with a remix of feelings and a sense of relief that his stint lasted only thirty-three days. "You wouldn't believe what went on there," he told a colleague. "I was sidetracked," he said to me years later, declining to speak about his Biscuit duties. After his stint with MI, he was reassigned to the work he'd prepared for, with a combat stress control team. Upon his return home from Iraq, he found his way back to the role he'd first trained for, as a child psychiatrist, caring for children with parents on active duty. Meanwhile, the ethical quandaries he faced at Abu Ghraib remained literally unspeakable. Told to keep his Biscuit service secret, he pulled out of a scheduled October 2004 panel discussion at a high-profile conference on psychiatry and law. He made a point of avoiding conversations with civilian colleagues if he sensed any risk that the subject would come up. Senior military colleagues advised him to do so; any hint of doubt or dissent in a junior officer's record could ruin his prospects for promotion, ending his career.

On April 28, 2004, Abu Ghraib became a household word. The CBS News program *60 Minutes II* broadcast the photos that became iconic. Nude men stacked like cordwood, a detainee nicknamed "Gus" on a leash, and a shrouded prisoner perched precariously on a cardboard box, wires tied to his fingers, transformed the politics of the Iraq war and the image of America. More grotesque images, some on videotape, were never released. Eleven military police guards were eventually convicted for bringing to life their perverse sexual imaginings.

Amid the chaos of Abu Ghraib, sadistic excess became the norm. Insurgents' mortar shells landed almost daily, killing and maiming soldiers and prisoners. Detainees rioted, sometimes using smuggled weapons. Bedlam begat boundary transgressions—some were necessary, even heroic; others rose to the level of atrocity. In the medical clinic, desperately short of staff and supplies, physicians' assistants amputated limbs, a dentist did heart surgery, and nurses took chest tubes from the dead for reuse.[4] And in the cell blocks, the stripping, shackling, and stress positions ordered up by interrogators devolved, in *Lord of the Flies* fashion, into madness—on Scott Uithol's watch. He would later be blamed by some for fomenting the madness—for being one of "America's torture doctors,"[5] in the words of a prominent medical ethicist who published a j'accuse against military medicine after the photos emerged. The irony behind this portrayal is that Abu Ghraib wouldn't have become a household word had Uithol been able to impose the tight control his superiors envisioned.

Beginnings: Toward a Science of Interrogation

The interrogation strategy that went awry at Abu Ghraib dates back a half-century, to Americans' alarm over "brainwashing" by communist interrogators. Accounts of forced conversions of wayward Chinese during the early months of Maoist rule were soon followed by the broadcast "confessions" of captured U.S. pilots. Airmen downed during the Korean War were taken across the Yalu River to China, where dozens "admitted" on tape to having committed war crimes. More than two-thirds of the 7,000 U.S. servicemen held by the Chinese either signed statements urging America to quit the conflict or "confessed" to sundry wrongdoings. The American public—and the military and intelligence communities— reacted with shock and embarrassment. Eminent researchers, including the psychologist Irving Janis, warned that the communists were employing drugs, hypnosis, and shock treatments to reorganize minds and induce trances. Novelists and filmmakers embellished the possibilities, imagining brainwashing techniques capable of turning people into robotic agents able to overthrow governments or kill their leaders.

Within the intelligence community, concern grew over the possibility that America's enemies had developed a scientific method for breaking prisoners' spirits. CIA director Allan Dulles turned to medicine for help. He engaged a Cornell neurologist, Harold Wolff, to investigate Maoist and Soviet counterresistance techniques.[6] The CIA and the Defense Department gave Dr. Wolff extraordinary access to former Soviet and Chinese interrogators, ex-POWs, and still-classified sources. Other researchers joined in the effort: the army engaged psychiatrist Robert Lifton and the air force enlisted sociologist Albert Biderman. They sought to reconstruct the methods used, to better grasp what these methods could and couldn't accomplish and to understand how and why they worked. CIA and military leaders had both offensive and defensive purposes in mind. They were intent on catching up with the communists in the race to develop more powerful counterresistance techniques, and they wanted to better prepare Americans for the possibility of capture by foes with contempt for the laws of war.

The conclusions from this crash program of inquiry into communist methods were more prosaic than many expected. Chinese and Soviet interrogators didn't use drugs or hypnosis, nor were they steered by Pavlovian mental programmers or other mad scientists of the sort imagined on Hollywood sets.

Some of their tactics were centuries old, dating back to the Inquisition and passed down since as a kind of torturers' lore. But the tactics weren't "torture" as most people imagine it. There were no thumbscrews, racks, bamboo splinters, or other devices for inflicting agony. Beatings were common, but interrogators rarely meted out lasting physical pain. To the contrary, they avoided face-to-face contests of physical endurance between themselves and the men they tried to break. Instead, they set these men against themselves—by, for example, forcing them to sit or stand in awkward positions that became excruciating over time. "The immediate source of pain," Biderman wrote, "is not the interrogator but the victim himself. . . . The motivational strength of the individual is likely to exhaust itself in this internal encounter."[7]

Invoking different models and metaphors, Wolff and others converged on similar understandings of what our foes did to soften their captives' minds. In the first phase, they found, those in charge took total command of each captive's environment, dictating minutia like the length of bathroom breaks and body positioning while sitting or standing. Prolonged isolation, flavorless food, confinement in tiny spaces, and extended darkness (or bright light) achieved what Biderman called "monopolization of perception." Sleep deprivation, loud noise, frigid temperatures, and disruption of daily routines wore down detainees. Small gestures of contempt—facial slaps and frequent insults—humiliated them. Threats fed fear and dependence. Filthy living conditions and lack of privacy further degraded them.

Under such conditions, Wolff and the others concluded, hopelessness and despair could take hold within weeks. These states of mind set the stage for the next phase: motivating captives to comply. To this end, the interrogator established an aura of omnipotence. For prolonged periods, he was his prisoner's sole human connection, with monopoly power to praise, punish, coax, scold, and reward. Rapport with the interrogator offered the only escape from despair. This opened possibilities for the sculpting of behavior and belief. Chinese and Soviet interrogators employed this strategy with an eye toward winning "confessions" of political error. Compliance, though, could take other forms. A half-century later, critics of the interrogation tactics employed at Abu Ghraib would neglect Biderman's distinction between "inducing" and "shaping" compliance. The Chinese and Soviets "shaped" compliance by rewarding sham confessions. But interrogators could, in theory, pursue other behavior-shaping goals, including getting prisoners to tell the truth.

By the late 1950s, CIA-sponsored physician-researchers were pursuing this possibility with fervor. Just because the communists hadn't used hypnosis, psychotropic drugs, or shock treatments didn't mean that our side couldn't give these and other technologies a try. We did so—on unwitting subjects—in a series of CIA-funded experiments that began during the Korean War and lasted until 1963. In the most notorious of these, Ewen Cameron, a Scotsman turned Canadian who climbed the academic ranks to become one of the most distinguished psychiatrists of his day, combined frequent, high-voltage shocks with weeks-long, drug-induced sleep to "de-pattern" the minds of mental patients. Dr. Cameron's avowed aim was to cure schizophrenia by wiping out deranged patterns of thinking, then refashioning patients' minds along healthier lines. To this end, he pressed ahead with shock treatments and drugged sleep until his patients became confused about time and place and unable to remember the past, to the point that they spoke only of their immediate bodily needs.

Only then did he try to reorder their minds, employing a strategy he called "psychic driving." For weeks, his stuporous patients listened, sixteen hours a day, every day, to tape loops condemning them for life failures they'd admitted in earlier interviews. Author John Marks[8] gives one example—a loop played to a thirty-year-old woman whose husband brought her to Dr. Cameron after she'd suffered a nervous breakdown:

Madeleine, you let your mother and father treat you as a child all through your single life. You let your mother check you up sexually after every date you had with a boy. . . . You never stood up for yourself. . . . They used to call you "crying Madeleine." Now that you have two children, you don't seem to be able to manage them and keep a good relationship with your husband. You are drifting apart. You don't go out together. You have not been able to keep him interested sexually.[9]

After a few or more weeks of such material, Dr. Cameron switched to a positive message:

> You mean to get well. To do this you must let your feelings come out. It is
> all right to express your anger. . . . You want to stop your mother bossing
> you around. Begin to assert yourself first in little things and soon you will
> be able to meet her on an equal basis. You will then be free to be a wife and
> mother just like other women.[10]

The obvious resemblance between Cameron's high-voltage (figuratively and literally) approach and communist detention regimens as reconstructed by Wolff and others caught the notice of a CIA psychologist, John Gittinger, in 1956. Cameron had developed depatterning and psychic driving as therapies. But in 1957, the CIA offered to fund his work. He embraced the opportunity, adding prolonged sensory deprivation to his depatterning regimen and trying LSD on some patients to augment their psychic driving experiences. For the next several years, the agency pursued an expanding array of research protocols aimed at enhancing the basic interrogation strategy it had reverse-engineered from studies of Chinese and Soviet methods. CIA researchers hired prostitutes to sneak LSD to clients, experimented with extracts from Amazon plants, and developed novel methods to make sensory deprivation nearly complete. A few subjects died under murky circumstances.[11] The CIA's Technical Services Division supported more than a hundred researchers at scores of institutions, managing to keep this funding mostly secret. Cameron's work, though, came the closest to achieving the agency's goal: a high-tech approach to "inducing" and "shaping" compliance.

By the early 1960s, though, CIA officials had given up on this goal. Neither Cameron nor others had figured out how to ensure that dazed, disoriented, dependent prisoners told interrogators the truth. The agency's research portfolio, moreover, came under scathing internal criticism in a 1963 report by the CIA inspector general, who warned that it put "the rights and interests of all Americans in jeopardy" and breached the medical ethics proscription against nontherapeutic "manipulation of human behavior."[12] The CIA officially suspended the program (though some claim it continued in diminished fashion for another decade[13]). When, in 1975, the program became public, as did its internal moniker, MK-ULTRA, a name the cleverest conspiracy theorist couldn't have dreamt up, vast numbers of Americans reacted with astonishment.

By then, the CIA had long since moved on. After the embarrassing disclosures of 1975, the agency abandoned its sponsorship of scientific efforts to improve on Soviet and Chinese interrogation methods. There were reports, though, that agency operatives taught harsh methods to Latin American militaries well into the 1980s.[14] And there were allegations that military dictatorships in Argentina, Chile, Uruguay, Guatemala, and elsewhere put these lessons to use to torture their opponents.[15] CIA training manuals from this period[16] tracked the model Wolff and his colleagues had constructed a generation before. They referenced psychoactive substances and even hypnosis as tools for bringing about the dependent state of mind necessary to "cause capitulation," and they endorsed "silent administration"—euphemistic for drugging subjects on the sly.[17] But they also warned of the unreliability of information so obtained. People can lie while under hypnosis, the authors noted. And drugs can cause hallucinations, delusions, and other alterations of belief, grossly distorting interrogators' results.

The most influential of these manuals, known as *Kubark Counterintelligence Interrogation,*[18] held that physicians were essential. So was teamwork between doctor and interrogator:

> The effect of most drugs depends more upon the personality of the subject than upon the physical characteristics of the drugs themselves. If the approval of Headquarters has been obtained and if a doctor is at hand for administration, one of the most important of the interrogator's functions is providing the doctor with a full and accurate description of the psychological make-up of the interrogatee, to facilitate the best possible choice of a drug.[19]

"The judicious choice of a drug with minimal side effects, its matching to the subject's personality, careful gauging of dosage, and a sense of timing" were vital to ensure that its "silent administration" went undetected by the subject. The effects of drugs given covertly would be "compelling to the subject since the perceived sensations originate entirely within himself." The doctor's "sense of timing" was also key to reducing the risk that drugs would elicit false information. "Their function is to cause capitulation, to aid in the shift from resistance to cooperation," the Kubark authors explained. "Once this shift has been accomplished," use of "coercive techniques," including psychoactive substances, "should be abandoned."[20] Thus the purpose of the drugs was to *motivate compliance,* not to *shape behavior.* The interrogator would shape behavior after resistance had been broken.

The various manuals made no reference to medical ethics qualms about this emphatically non-therapeutic work. And when the manuals became public after the Clinton administration declassified them in 1997, the press paid no attention to these qualms—or to the close match between the Kubark theory of interrogation and the model reverse-engineered from studies of Chinese and Soviet methods forty years before. The ensuing political furor centered on foreign policy: The manuals and other newly disclosed materials made it plain that the United States had taught counterinsurgency tactics widely seen as torture to thousands of Central and South Americans during the Reagan years.[21] The CIA stopped doing so in 1986, as reports of human rights abuses in Latin America mounted.[22] Thereafter, the agency's facility with Kubark methods atrophied quickly, according to psychologists and psychiatrists in the national security community with whom I've spoken. Institutional memory ebbed as those familiar with these methods (and capable of employing them) quit or retired. By the time of the 9/11 attacks, the CIA's capabilities in this realm were a thing of the past. They became so without any official verdict—from the CIA, its congressional overseers, or professional bodies—concerning the propriety of medical involvement of the sort Kubark required.

Learning from the Enemy: The "Pre-academic Laboratory"

But the model that Wolff, Biderman, and their colleagues had constructed persisted in another setting. "Confessions" by downed pilots taken prisoner in North Korea shocked the air force into developing a training program for personnel at risk of capture. The army and navy would follow suit. The program, which became known as SERE (survival, evasion, resistance, and escape), aimed to prepare participants for ill treatment of the sort endured by American POWs in Korea. To this end, the air force relied on the Wolff-Biderman model to reverse-engineer the enemy's methods. Trainees spent weeks in the wilderness eating bugs, eluding pursuers, and otherwise honing survival skills. After they were "captured," they were held in mock prison camps and subjected to assorted abuses.

Clinical psychologists oversaw and sequenced these abuses, including sleep deprivation, exposure to cold temperatures, prolonged standing in painful positions, and confinement in tiny spaces. But whereas Wolff and Biderman had outlined a process for reducing prisoners to despair, the "pre-academic laboratory" (Pentagon-speak for the mock POW experience) was designed to build trainees' confidence. The idea was to push trainees to the edge, but not over it, to boost their resistance. "The [mock] interrogator must recognize when a student is overly frustrated and doing a poor job resisting," a SERE school operating manual warned. "At this point the interrogator must temporarily back off."[23] To this end, psychologists watched trainees closely, stopping the water-dousing or forced standing when stress seemed to overwhelm them.

That the psychologists sought to build resistance, not to break it, is underscored by an internal battle over waterboarding's place in the curriculum. By 2007, only the navy's SERE school still included it—a bow to fliers who'd been waterboarded while captive in Vietnam. It was "an emotional issue with former Navy POWs," a SERE official observed.[24] "Nostalgia," a former SERE psychologist told me less sympathetically. In 2007, the interservice agency that oversees SERE acted to drop it. "[T]he water board should not be used," agency officials told navy and Marine Corps commanders. "[I]t leaves students psychologically defeated with no ability to resist under pressure. Once a student is taught that they can be beaten, and there is no way to resist, it is difficult to develop psychological hardiness."[25]

The power of the waterboard to teach hopelessness arises from the biology of suffocation: Water is poured over a cloth that covers the trainee's nose and

mouth. This creates an airtight seal, making it impossible to inhale. This sensation triggers reflexive terror. Subjects gasp and flail about. The mind is useless as
a defense. Trainees know that it's just an exercise and that their "interrogators"
will remove the soaked cloth in seconds. Yet they experience drowning and think
they will die. The craving for air overpowers all. The waterboard, wrote chief
SERE psychologist Gary Percival, thus "risks promoting learned helplessness."

Percival's concern about learned helplessness reflected SERE training
doctrine. "Maximum effort will be made to ensure that students do not develop a sense of 'learned helplessness' during the pre-academic laboratory,"[26]
a 2002 training manual stated. Use of this term in a training manual constituted a conceptual leap beyond the Wolff-Biderman model. SERE psychologists had embraced a clinical theory of despair, built upon behavioral psychologist Martin Seligman's 1960s experiments with dogs exposed to electric
shocks. Seligman caged and shocked his animals under varying conditions:
Some could escape (by moving to a safe area) or stop the shocks (by pressing
a lever); others could do nothing to discontinue them or make them less frequent. The unlucky creatures in the latter group typically stopped trying, to
the point that they made no efforts to escape even when moved to a setting
that offered them a way out.[27]

Seligman coined the term "learned helplessness" to capture this phenom-
enon, and he promoted it as a way to think about how people become depressed. Psychiatrists seized on this idea, and Dr. Seligman became famous, as
both a behavioral science pioneer and a guru of positive thinking. He authored
best-selling books with such titles as *Learned Optimism, The Optimistic Child,*
and *Authentic Happiness*[28] and in the 1990s became recognized as a preeminent
figure in the treatment of depression. People develop depression, Seligman and
his followers hold, when they come to believe they can do nothing about the
bad that comes their way. Inveterate optimists have the best odds for averting
depression, but pessimists can protect themselves, by resisting their own can't-
do thoughts as they arise. And for the already-depressed, psychotherapy should
have a simple aim: persuade patients to believe there's a way out even when
things look bleak, and they'll break out of their dysphoric funks. To this end,
psychologists and psychiatrists developed what they called cognitive behavioral

therapy (CBT), aimed at reframing people's understandings of life's possibilities in more positive terms. Studies of CBT's efficacy found it did better than
other treatments.[29] People who move from "I can't do anything right" toward
belief that they can shape their own fates become more hopeful and otherwise
less symptomatic. CBT also proved effective against anxiety disorders, including posttraumatic stress disorder.

SERE psychologists took notice. They reimagined resistance training as
a total-immersion variant of CBT. Just as cognitive therapists verbally escort-
ed their patients through bad memories (and even, at times, took patients on
location to reenact stressful experiences), SERE trainers guided "students"
through sequences of abuse, with an eye toward growing their belief in their
capacity to cope. "Consider everything the enemy does as a technique," navy
command psychologist Bryce Lefever told me in November 2009, recalling
his days as a SERE trainer. "You are less likely to be taken in by it. . . . They
are going to try to destroy your hope, they are going to threaten you with
death, they are going to make you miserable. . . . Our job was to expose them
to all these techniques so they could say, 'Oh, yeah, I really fell for that. I'm
going to do better next time.'"

Psychiatrists call this stress inoculation, a term SERE's designers embraced. At their annual meetings each spring, SERE psychologists focused on
the study of resilience. All of this happened behind high walls: The SERE
program is classified, ostensibly to keep enemies from outwitting it. As a result,
SERE psychologists could neither publish their thinking nor bring in outside
colleagues to critique it. Isolated from their peers, they created a parallel professional universe, rotating among SERE schools, clinical care, and support for
Special Forces. They sometimes went on special-ops missions, rappelling from
helicopters and advising on battlefield deception. "Some of these guys were op
docs—SEAL wannabes," a former navy psychologist told me. They breathed
in the special-ops culture of audacity and segregated themselves from their
closest civilian counterparts—psychologists and psychiatrists who consult to
criminal investigators and practice in prison settings.

This separation had consequences—for their career chances and their
understanding of interrogation. Doctors who serve in the armed forces

follow a more or less standard career trajectory—twenty years, or a little more, during which they rise to the rank of colonel or lieutenant colonel (in the army and air force) or captain (in the navy). They then "retire" in their forties or fifties (with pensions in excess of 40 percent of their final pay) to lucrative civilian jobs. But SERE psychologists had a rougher time of it. Special-ops derring-do didn't translate into civilian opportunities. Neither did knowledge of the cognitive psychology of torture. It was as if police departments, private investigators, and other civilian employers had posted signs saying, "No SERE alumni need apply."

Some SERE alums marketed their training methods to multinational corporations, offering to prepare at-risk executives to handle hostage takers. But others saw broader possibilities. They came to believe that torture, or something close to it, could extract truth, if well-planned. "We all knew from experience," said Dr. Lefever, "that these techniques, these SERE training techniques, were pretty effective not only at training but . . . at exposing vulnerabilities in our own students." Before they were taken "prisoner," trainees were given mock secrets to keep. Routinely, they failed. "It was a kind of astonishing thing," Lefever recalled. "You could have truly brave American patriots, even in a training setting, talking rather freely about stuff they shouldn't have been talking about."

In the wake of revelations about abusive, post-9/11 interrogation practices at Guantanamo and Abu Ghraib—practices that mimed SERE methods—political liberals, including myself, preferred to believe that these practices didn't "work"—that they didn't draw out accurate information. But a body of evidence, mostly classified, supports Lefever's claim that SERE methods *can* extract truth in training settings, even though trainees know that their captivity isn't real.

"Voodoo Science?"

This possibility intrigued James "Jim" Mitchell, SERE's chief psychologist for much of the 1990s. When Mitchell retired from the air force in May 2001, he set about becoming a resistance training entrepreneur. He created companies and hired former military colleagues to market his mix of clinical knowhow and special-ops daring. He had no shortage of self-confidence: He'd joined the air force out of high school in 1974, learned to defuse bombs, gone to college while on active duty, then collected a PhD in psychology.[30] Stress management seized his interest early on. It was essential to his work as a bomb disposal tech and central to his doctoral thesis on behavioral approaches to high blood pressure. And he took an interest in Seligman's ideas and their potential for empowering people to cope with dire circumstances.

The world of SERE and special ops was a perfect match for Mitchell's mix of machismo and behavioral science background. And his charisma and networking skills were just as good a match for the business of seeking corporate and government contracts. He offered himself as a scientist—and as a bridge between cutting-edge research and real-world needs. Preparing executives to handle hostage situations, assessing the reliability of informants, and getting reluctant sources to talk were among the services his several firms offered. He made the science seem simple to potential clients with no patience for academics' "on the other hand" reservations.

Among some in the SERE and special-ops communities, Mitchell's marketing pitch aroused concern. "Jim says he's a scientist, but he's not a scientist," a prominent physician and SERE researcher told me. "The Mitchell that I met in the past was usually someone who said 'I know.' . . . Every time you'd ask him a question, he'd look impatient and irritable. He didn't enjoy being questioned about data."

When nineteen hijackers seized four planes and killed more than 3,000 people, Mitchell's moment came. Within weeks of the 9/11 attacks, the CIA and Special Forces were collecting captives—and close to clueless about how to get reliable information from them. No research decisively answered the question of which interrogation techniques "work." Nor could it have, since research of this sort is both unethical and barred by international law. The Nuremberg Code, promulgated in 1947 by the court that condemned seven Nazi doctors to die, forbade research on human subjects without their consent.[31] So have multiple treaties, regulations, and codes of ethics since. CIA and military interrogators were thus left with their hunches and traditions.

An army field manual offered some guidance on how to manipulate emotions and build rapport within the confines of the Geneva Conventions.[32] New enlistees—typically teenagers without college experience—could become interrogators by taking a several-week course at the Army Intelligence Center in Fort Huachuca, Arizona. They learned to show kindness, feign empathy, flatter, and shame—and to exploit contradictions and come up with clever ruses. In tents and shacks at Bagram, Kandahar, and other sites across Afghanistan, anecdotes became "knowledge" as interrogators swapped stories about prisoners whose language they didn't speak and whose politics they didn't understand. "Interrogation doctrine in this country is based on old wives' tales," a high-ranking military intelligence specialist told me in a 2009 interview, recalling his work with interrogators in Afghanistan and, later, Iraq. "They come out of the booth and say: 'Oh, that was effective.' But how do they know—compared to what?"

In 9/11's immediate wake, effectiveness was an urgent matter. War against spectral extremists and their networks required pinpoint intelligence—about plans, capabilities, and personal relationships. In World War II, Korea, the first Gulf War, and even Vietnam, interrogation was peripheral; massive firepower and the technology to deliver it mattered more. But in Afghanistan and across the webs and warrens of jihadist fanaticism from Europe to the Philippines, interrogation was central. And fear of another cataclysm like 9/11, or worse, kept the CIA and military focused on the task of extracting maximum information from captives who might harbor pieces of the puzzle. At the CIA's McLean, Virginia headquarters, though, expertise on how to interrogate anyone, let alone Islamic fundamentalists, was lacking. As agency operatives, special-ops soldiers, and their Afghan allies-of-convenience took territory and prisoners, Counter-Terrorism Center chief Cofer Black cast about for interrogation solutions. That's when a former Veterans Administration psychologist, Kirk M. Hubbard, redirected the course of America's post-9/11 campaign against terror.

More than a decade earlier, Hubbard had made an unusual career switch, from clinical practice at the Hampton, Virginia VA Medical Center to a job at the CIA, supporting clandestine operations overseas. He served in Tokyo, London, and possibly elsewhere, impressing superiors with his savvy. By 9/11, he'd done stints back at headquarters for a unit whose existence remains secret, the Operational Assessment Division (OAD). His opaque OAD job titles, Chief of Operations, then Chief of the Research and Analysis Branch, reveal little about his responsibilities beyond the hint that he had an important role in assessing clandestine activities. But the contacts he forged with mental health professionals working in national security convey his main interest: bringing behavioral science to the front lines of the fight against terror.

Hubbard's position at the CIA gave him the chance to do so. Paramilitary teams run by the agency's Directorate of Operations worked closely with army, navy, and air force special operations units. Hubbard became part of an informal network of military and civilian psychologists and psychiatrists with shared interests in psyops, Special Forces selection, resistance training, and the reliability of "humint" (human intelligence). He wasn't a SERE psychologist, but he went to their professional meetings. He wasn't a research scientist, but he was inveterately curious—open to fresh ideas and disinclined to stay within bureaucratic silos. How he came to meet Jim Mitchell remains unclear. What's certain, though, is that Hubbard came to see the challenge of extracting humint from hostile prisoners Mitchell's way.

Thanks to superb reporting by Scott Shane, Mark Benjamin, and Katherine Eban, the fact that Mitchell personally waterboarded several Al Qaeda detainees held by the CIA is widely known. So is the fact that Mitchell drew on his SERE experience to design regimens to break these detainees. Mitchell "reverse-engineered" SERE, the story goes, without regard for common knowledge that torture doesn't work. He was a rogue operator—a practitioner of "voodoo science"[33]—who somehow wheedled the CIA into allowing him to have his way with its captives. I helped to tell this story, in articles I wrote (with British human-rights lawyer Jonathan Marks) for the *New England Journal of Medicine* and the *New York Times*.

But the story is incomplete. It's indeed common wisdom among political progressives that torture doesn't work—if, by "work," we mean extraction of accurate information from hostile informants. Miming communist interrogation methods, Marks and I wrote in 2005, yields compliance of a mindless sort: People being abused to the breaking point will say anything to get the torture to stop. This makes torture a powerful tool for extracting false confessions (once you break your victim, you need only provide the script) but a poor means for seeking truth, since the truth might differ from what the victim figures his torturer wants to hear.[34]

From a human rights perspective, this is a nice, win-win story: Avoid torture (or anything approaching it) and you'll get *better* information from reluctant interviewees. But this story overlooks a point Albert Biderman made fifty years earlier. If well designed and strategically sequenced to reduce captives to despair, the abuses he cataloged could "induce" a compliant state of mind. But the "shaping" of compliant behavior was another matter. It turned on the interrogator's perceived omnipotence—his monopoly power to punish and reward. He could use this power as the Chinese and Soviets did, to extract false confessions. But he could also use it to force fearful and hopeless prisoners to tell the truth—if he could detect falsehoods in real time and punish them swiftly.

SERE psychologists grasped this latter possibility. They'd seen it play out as American soldiers spilled "secrets" under the pressures of the "pre-academic laboratory." Like Bryce Lefever, Jim Mitchell believed that the stressors they'd designed to inoculate trainees against torture could be re-mixed—and enhanced—to extract lifesaving intelligence from actors intent on doing Americans harm. But the breaking of prisoners, by itself, wouldn't be enough. Biderman's insight here was critical. The interrogator would need to shape the behavior of the men he broke by distinguishing truth from invention, then rewarding the former.

Kirk Hubbard became convinced that this model could deliver better results, more quickly, than the "rapport-building" techniques used by law enforcement agencies. It was science *based*—grounded in Wolff's, Biderman's, and Seligman's work—albeit not scientifically *proven*. In the weeks after 9/11, as the White House and CIA sought frantically to prevent the next attack, Hubbard arranged for Jim Mitchell to meet with CIA leadership. "I didn't make the decision to hire them," Hubbard told me in an e-mail about the roles played by Mitchell and John "Bruce" Jessen (a former SERE colleague who would become Mitchell's partner). "I just introduced them as potential assets."[35]

The CIA Buys In

Within the CIA, Hubbard had to reckon with a rival. Psychologist R. Scott Shumate—trained, like Hubbard, as a therapist—had for years worked in support of clandestine operations overseas. A 2005 bio blurb, prepared by Shumate to promote his candidacy for an American Psychological Association committee, boasted of his "extensive experience and knowledge of Middle Eastern culture" and service "under highly stressful and difficult circumstances."[36] He claimed credit for having "interviewed many renowned individuals associated with various terrorist networks" and said he'd served as "the chief operational psychologist for the [CIA] Counter-Terrorism Center."

Shumate would later tell colleagues in the national security community that he'd objected to Mitchell's methods, warning that his approach was ethically dubious and unlikely to work. But according to Hubbard, Shumate's pushback was self-serving: "Scott saw himself as the chief psychologist in CTC and was very protective of 'his turf' . . . [H]e wanted to control (if possible) psychology in CTC, or at least be a part of it if could not control it [sic]." What, exactly, Shumate had in mind as an alternative to Mitchell's "enhanced" interrogation strategy remains uncertain. What's clear is that Shumate lost out—within CTC, then within the CIA as a whole. "He simply wasn't a player in CTC when it came to the interrogation program," Hubbard said. "He was in way over his head, I believe. I think he truly believes that he objected to the EITs [enhanced interrogation techniques] on moral or ethical grounds, but I think there is much more to it than that."

When, exactly, CTC director Cofer Black and CIA director George Tenet decided to go with Mitchell is unclear. But by December 2001, Mitchell and Hubbard had won out. As the CIA inspector general reported in 2004 (in a "Special Review" of "Counterterrorism Detention and Interrogation

Activities" that wasn't declassified until 2009), the agency gave Mitchell the nod to prepare a report on how to counter Al Qaeda's interrogation resistance techniques.[37] Mitchell enlisted Bruce Jessen as his coauthor. This decision would prove momentous. Jessen brought little to the partnership by way of new ideas. But he was still on active duty as the senior SERE psychologist at the Joint Personnel Recovery Agency (JPRA), a Spokane, Washington–based unit that oversaw army, navy, and air force resistance training. Jessen could, and did, tap into JPRA and the services' SERE schools for information about the physical and psychological effects of isolation, waterboarding, and other stressors. More important, he could, and later would, use JPRA as a platform to promote "enhanced" interrogation methods to U.S. commanders around the world.

Mitchell and Jessen rushed their project to completion. By February 12, 2002, they'd written a paper, "Recognizing and Developing Countermeasures to Al-Qa'ida Resistance to Interrogation Techniques: A Resistance Training Perspective." Not only did CIA leadership embrace the Mitchell-Jessen approach; the agency asked JPRA to arrange training in SERE methods for interrogators in Afghanistan and Guantanamo Bay. In his capacity as JPRA's SERE psychologist, Jessen did so. JPRA's chief, meanwhile, sent Mitchell's and Jessen's paper to top army, navy, and air force commanders, urging them to look to SERE for help in extracting information from hostile detainees. "After over 30 years of training," he offered, "we have become quite proficient with both specialized resistance and the ways to defeat it."[38] The idea of using SERE stressors to break prisoners' resistance spread to commanders in every theater, including Afghanistan and Guantanamo Bay.

But Mitchell took the idea to its farthest extreme, on the CIA's behalf. How, exactly, he understood the ethics of tapping his clinical and behavioral science background to reduce prisoners to despair remains unknown.[39] But Hubbard's understanding is clear. In an unpublished commentary he shared with me, he rejected the relevance of clinical ethics, including the "do no harm" ideal, to psychologists and physicians "not serving in a doctor/patient role." Doctors, he said, owe it to their country to become involved:

What does seem unethical is for psychologists/psychiatrists to not use our knowledge of human behavior to assist in preventing terrorist threats to innocent victims or to our Western democratic way of life. I reject the notion that it is somehow unethical to put the lives of innocent Americans ahead of the interests of Islamic terrorists. . . . I think each of us has an obligation to try to balance the law, our duty to our fellow citizens, and [the] ethical codes of our professional organizations. For me, this balance favors society over the so-called rights of terrorists.

The limits that mattered for Hubbard and Mitchell were those that U.S. law imposed—in particular, federal statutes banning torture. Hubbard's interrogators would need a legal safe harbor—a definition of "torture" sufficiently capacious to allow Mitchell to take his methods into the field. So, in the late winter and early spring of 2002, the agency set about constructing one. CIA officials consulted with psychologists, psychiatrists, and others in academia and the military, looking to make the "enhanced" approach more effective and to build support for their claim that it didn't constitute "torture."

Early on, they tapped JPRA for both purposes. By early March, Jessen had developed slide presentations, titled "Al Qaeda Resistance Contingency Training" and "Exploitation," setting out a strategy for extracting information from uncooperative prisoners. These presentations included slides on "isolation and degradation," "sensory deprivation," "physiological pressures" (a SERE euphemism for beatings and other physical abuse) and "psychological pressures."[40]

JPRA also assembled findings on the mental health effects of resistance training—findings that backed SERE psychologists' claim that it strengthened students' coping skills. Bush administration legal policy makers would later invoke these findings as evidence that "enhanced" interrogation wasn't torture.[41] SERE training, according to JPRA, had negligible psychiatric side effects in the elite war-fighters selected to receive it. SERE methods thus wouldn't cause "severe mental pain or suffering"—the law's test for psychological torture—when used to break terror suspects' resistance.

Hubbard embraced this proposition, ignoring the critical difference between resistance training and use of SERE methods to crack resistance. SERE training built resistance, with minimal mental health side effects, because psychologists took care to avoid inducing a sense of helplessness. Jessen and Mitchell, though, made learned helplessness their goal. SERE trainers' success at avoiding psychiatric sequelae was thus beside the point. Mitchell's method could succeed only by inflicting mental suffering—suffering "severe" enough to bring on learned helplessness.

Mitchell and Hubbard also consulted with Martin Seligman. In December 2001, according to Scott Shane of the *New York Times,* Seligman hosted the two (along with others) at his suburban Philadelphia home.[42] Did Seligman advise Mitchell or Hubbard on how to employ learned helplessness to break prisoners' resistance? His denials have been emphatic. "I am grieved and horrified," he wrote in a short memo he sent me, "that good science, which has helped so many people overcome depression, may have been used for such dubious purposes." He acknowledged only that he spoke on learned helplessness at a JPRA meeting in May 2002 and that Mitchell and Jessen were in the audience:

> I was invited to speak about how American . . . personnel could use what is known about learned helplessness to resist torture and evade successful interrogation by their captors. This is what I spoke about.

Seligman added:

> I have had no professional contact with Jessen and Mitchell since then. I have never worked under government contract (or any other contract) on any aspect of torture, nor would I be willing to do work on torture. I have never worked on interrogation; I have never seen an interrogation and I have only a passing knowledge of the literature on interrogation.

But sometime in the spring of 2002, according to a CIA source, Seligman met with Mitchell, Jessen, and Hubbard in Philadelphia. "The fact that we had a meeting in Philadelphia," said the source, a meeting participant, "means that Mitchell/Jessen were at least thinking about interrogation strategies." Seligman wanted to help and understood what Mitchell had in mind. But having built his reputation as a clinical pioneer—the man who'd discovered learned helplessness, then transformed depressed people's lives through "learned optimism"—he didn't want to be seen as telling CIA operatives how to break people by inducing despair. So he walked a careful line, keeping to the question of what the science did and didn't support while abstaining from how-to advice. Seligman, said the CIA source, had a "classic approach-avoidance conflict regarding helping us."

Parsing Seligman's denials leads to the conclusion that he feinted left but didn't lie.[43] He declined an interview, which made follow-up questions difficult. But when I asked him (by e-mail) whether Mitchell and Jessen had acted unethically by turning learned helplessness theory toward the task of breaking terror suspects,[44] he responded: "I went to a college whose motto was, 'Princeton in the nation's service.' I admired Gen. [George] Casey's quote of Isaiah at the Ft. Hood service [for victims of the Fort Hood massacre]: 'Who will answer the call? Whom shall I send? Here am I. Send me.'"

Going Live

By the time of the Philadelphia meeting, CIA preparations for "enhanced" interrogation had reached high intensity, energized by what looked like an extraordinary opportunity. At 2 AM on March 28, a Pakistani SWAT team seized Abu Zubaydah, a Saudi whom some at the CIA thought was Al Qaeda's third in command. Top CIA officials convinced themselves—and told the president—that Zubaydah harbored a trove of information about pending attacks and sleeper cells. Zubaydah, who barely survived horrific wounds,[45] was flown to a secret CIA site outside Bangkok. He was treated and then interrogated, initially by FBI agents who used conventional, "rapport-building" techniques. CIA officials, though, were sure Zubaydah was withholding details that could save thousands. So they decided to send Jim Mitchell to break him—if they could get the lawyers to go along.

Months would pass before final Justice Department approval for what Mitchell had in mind. But once approval seemed likely, CIA leadership made the call. Kirk Hubbard answered it, quite literally, on the way back from Philadelphia. "I received a phone call indicating 'they' wanted Mitchell to depart that night along with others from CTC," Hubbard remembers.[46] "Mitchell had about twelve hours' notice that he was being flown to meet AZ [Zubaydah]." Exactly when Mitchell began his brutish efforts with Zubaydah (and based on what sort of approval) remains a matter of dispute. An FBI interrogator who remained on the scene after Mitchell took charge alleged that Mitchell and his team engaged in "borderline torture" many weeks before the Justice Department's Office of Legal Counsel (OLC) gave its final okay in its notorious August 2002 "torture memos."[47] And much of the press coverage of Mitchell's activities casts him as a cowboy—a rogue player who disregarded limits set back in McLean. Not true, Hubbard insisted: "Jim Mitchell, et al. didn't take a pee without written approval from headquarters. . . . CIA leadership approved and is responsible for all that occurred. Mitchell & Jessen were not mavericks operating on their own."

What is clear—and remarkable—is that even as Mitchell served as maestro of the abuse that much of the world came to see as torture, he kept his clinical hat on, purporting to care for Abu Zubaydah's mental health. His doing so played a critical role in the development and spread of "enhanced" interrogation. His "psychological assessment" of Zubaydah, based on "direct interviews with and observations of the subject,"[48] gave the OLC cover to conclude that waterboarding wouldn't cause Zubaydah "severe mental pain or suffering." Later, it would shield the OLC's lawyers against charges of misconduct.

Mitchell's "assessment" was a series of claims, unmoored from evidence, about Zubaydah's "incredibly strong resolve" and hardiness under stress.[49] It was transparently designed to meet the needs of OLC's lawyers by lending clinical weight to their claim that Mitchell's remix of SERE methods wasn't torture. Zubaydah, he wrote, was "remarkably resilient," "ab[le] to manage his mood and emotions," and without known "history of mood disturbance or other psychiatric pathology." Mitchell marshaled no evidence to back these assertions. His "assessment" lacked the detailed reporting on mood, feelings, and thought processes necessary for a clinical evaluation to be of passable quality. He disregarded word from FBI and CIA analysts who had reviewed Zubaydah's diaries and found a tendency to collapse under stress.[50] Mitchell also ignored the possible effects of a severe head wound that Zubaydah had suffered in battle against the Soviets as a teen.

Circular Lawyering

Measured by conventional clinical standards, Mitchell's "assessment" was malpractice. But for the lawyers this didn't matter. Its clinical mien, not its medical science, gave the OLC the cover it sought. And more than seven years later, Mitchell's unsupported claims about Zubaydah's mental strength became a basis for the Justice Department's decision to absolve the torture memos' authors of professional misconduct. The department's ethics arm issued a finding of misconduct, based in part on the authors' misuse of JPRA data showing that SERE training posed minimal mental health risk.[51] The authors had claimed mental harm to Zubaydah was "highly improbable" since SERE students hadn't suffered it. But the ethics office at Justice said this assertion improperly overlooked the difference between use of SERE methods to build and to break resistance. True enough, said a top Justice official, but Mitchell's "individualized" assessment filled this analytic gap. It supported the conclusion that "mental health consequences" were "highly improbable." On this basis, the department threw out the misconduct finding against the torture memos' two authors, Jay Bybee (now a federal judge) and John Yoo (who parlayed the memos' notoriety into prominence as a conservative commentator).[52]

There was more than a bit of bootstrapping involved. The doctor and the lawyers relied on each other to justify practices that the rest of the world later saw as torture. Mitchell's "assessment," unhinged from fact, empowered the lawyers to make a case unhinged from law. His clinical credentials were enough—a substitute for facts, in the minds of attorneys who were supposed to reason tightly from facts. The lawyers' conclusions, in turn, shielded Mitchell from criminal accountability for what he did to Zubaydah and, later, others. And in the end, his "assessment" protected the lawyers from career-ending sanctions.

Physicians had an equally important role in the bootstrapping. By the time Yoo and Bybee gave their okay (orally in late July 2002, then in writing on August 1), CIA physicians were on hand with Mitchell at the Bangkok black site.[53] Yoo and Bybee conditioned their approval on the presence of a "medical expert with SERE experience," tasked with stopping the proceedings if "medically necessary to prevent severe mental or physical harm to Zubaydah."[54] "Medical necessity" had acquired a new meaning, outside the health insurance realm.

The physician in attendance played another, more pernicious role in the Yoo-Bybee legal design. To be a torturer in the eyes of the law, pain or suffering tantamount to torture isn't enough; "specific intent" to inflict the suffering is required. That means, in practice, that the suffering must be the torturer's *purpose;* knowledge that suffering might ensue isn't enough.[55] Yoo and Bybee seized this opening. Having a doctor on hand was key. The "constant presence of personnel with medical training who have the authority to stop the interrogation," they claimed, was enough to show absence of "specific intent" to inflict severe pain or suffering.[56] The presence of physicians proved "good faith"—an "honest belief" that severe pain or suffering wouldn't occur. The "honest belief" might be wrong, but this was beside the point: "Honest belief" was enough to show that committing torture didn't make one a torturer. Thus the doctors' mere presence guaranteed impunity, *whether or not* they protected Zubaydah from pain or suffering rising to the level of torture.

Handed this lawyerly carte blanche, Mitchell went to work with ferocity. Over the summer, Bruce Jessen joined him, leaving the air force to become a principal in Mitchell's firm. Meticulous records were kept, including detailed interrogation logs and ninety-two videos (all later destroyed) of encounters with Zubaydah. Physicians and other medical personnel observed the "enhanced" procedures and made notes.[57] A review by the CIA inspector general counted eighty-three waterboarding "applications"—that is, eighty-three separate simulated drownings. (By comparison, SERE trainees typically endured just one or two.)

Each application, moreover, went well beyond what SERE students experienced. In SERE training, a cloth was first draped over the student's eyes and forehead, then soaked with water from a small cup and lowered to cover the nose and mouth. To keep the cloth saturated (so as to make breathing difficult), the instructor added water for twenty to forty seconds; then the cloth was removed.[58] But according to the inspector general, Mitchell's team poured much more water—"large volumes." Mitchell and Jessen, said the inspector general, "acknowledged that the Agency's use of the technique differed from that used in SERE training [*sic*] and explained that the Agency's technique is different because it is 'for real' and is more poignant and convincing."

Scaling Up

Whether Mitchell's "alternative set of procedures," as President Bush later called them, extracted lifesaving intelligence from Zubaydah is a matter of fierce dispute. What's clear, though, is that word got around quickly within the national security establishment that Mitchell's methods *worked*. The false story spread that Zubaydah had agreed to tell all after only thirty-five seconds on the waterboard.[59] His interrogation became the prototype for a clandestine cottage industry. By the end of May 2005, the CIA was holding ninety-four terror suspects at "black sites" around the world and had subjected twenty-eight to Mitchell's methods.

Jessen himself developed the first "curriculum" for CIA interrogators.[60] His JPRA colleague, psychologist Gary Percival, led the first training session, on July 1–2, 2002. Percival and JPRA instructor Joseph Witsch explained and demonstrated "physical pressures," including waterboarding, to CIA officers preparing to deploy to Afghanistan and elsewhere.[61] By November 2002, the agency had its own two-week course, "designed to train, qualify, and certify individuals as agency interrogators." The "curriculum" included a week of classroom instruction, followed by a week of "'hands-on' training in EITs."[62] To perform EITs, certification was essential. The CIA had created a corps of operatives trained to torture,[63] pursuant to a plausible, science-based model.

"Medical" Procedures

As "enhanced" interrogation scaled up, medical involvement became integral, to the point that waterboarding, sleep deprivation, "walling,"[64] and other abuses were reinvented as medical procedures. Condemnation of the Yoo-Bybee memos, leaked in 2004,[65] occasioned this reinvention. In high-visibility fashion, the Bush administration withdrew the memos, backing away from their sweeping claims about the president's power to ignore the law. But a secret set of replacement memos insisted that Mitchell's methods weren't torture, so long as "medical personnel" helped to design them and oversaw their administration.[66]

To this end, CIA physicians reengineered waterboarding to make it "medically appropriate." They required that potable saline solution, not "plain water," be poured, to prevent detainees who drink it from developing hyponatremia—a dangerously low concentration of sodium in the blood. To guard against aspiration (inhalation of vomited food), they ordered that detainees be put on a liquid diet before waterboarding. And to respond to spasms of the larynx—life-threatening when they persist after water is poured—they mandated that tracheotomy equipment be on hand.[67] The CIA's Office of Medical Services (OMS), moreover, required that a physician be present to watch for respiratory distress, loss of consciousness, and other problems.[68] That such problems arose is strongly suggested by a warning in the OMS "Guidelines" for medical attendance at "enhanced" interrogations: "In our limited experience, extensive sustained use of the waterboard can introduce new risks."[69] OMS acknowledged in its "Guidelines" that it was conducting an experiment of sorts, noting that SERE students were typically waterboarded only once. To learn the most possible from this novel endeavor, OMS told its physicians, rigorous data collection was essential.

> In order to best inform future medical judgments and recommendations, it is important that every application of the waterboard be thoroughly documented: how long each application (and the entire procedure) lasted, how much water was used in the process (realizing that much splashes off), how exactly the water was applied, if a seal was achieved, if the naso- or oropharynx was filled, what sort of volume was expelled, how long was the break between applications, and how the subject looked between each treatment.[70]

Most of the CIA's medical judgments were less evidence based. Sleep deprivation of up to 180 hours, imposed by shackling and forced standing, was said not to "have significant physiological effects" aside from a "temporar[y]" impact on brain function.[71] This claim ignored growing evidence that sleep loss predisposes people to cardiovascular disease, cancer, diabetes, and infection as well as disorders of mood and thought.[72] And at the CIA's black sites, medical personnel who oversaw walling, stomach slaps, cold-water dousing, and other "procedures" were instructed to stop these when "medically appropriate"—as if clinical researchers had studied these procedures and developed science-based practice protocols. Physiological jargon—discussions of metabolic compensation for cold temperatures, avoidance of "extension-flexion injury" and bodily heat loss during immersion in frigid water[73]—masked the lack of scientific answers to questions that couldn't ethically be studied.

"To Do No Harm"

Incongruously, the OMS instructed doctors who oversaw interrogation that "[a]ll medical officers remain under the professional obligation to do no harm." This absurdist directive silenced conversation about the tension between Hippocratic ideals and what they were doing. It feigned uncompromising Hippocratic commitment, making it awkward for CIA doctors to admit that they were straying.

For the CIA's physicians, there were dodges aplenty: (1) the doctors *helped* detainees by making the "procedures" more humane; (2) they were "just following orders" (others made the decision to adopt the Mitchell model); and (3) they weren't acting as physicians—or, at least, as caregivers—and thus weren't bound by medical ethics. These dodges were disingenuous. Had the doctors not helped to plan and supervise "enhanced" interrogation, the CIA couldn't have gone ahead with it—the lawyers wouldn't have approved. And the "following orders" claim begs the question of the orders' propriety: The law requires CIA physicians to adhere to their profession's ethical obligations even when this means saying no to instructions from above. The proposition that the doctors weren't acting as physicians is a prevarication. Not only did they exercise clinical judgment, science based or otherwise; they intervened as caregivers, ordering a halt to "procedures" and providing treatment when injury ensued.

Physicians served a larger function in the CIA's black sites: They lent an aura of benevolence and restraint to a brutish endeavor. Bush administration lawyers tacitly acknowledged this in their memos by making medical involvement critical to their conclusion that enhanced interrogation wasn't torture. Physician involvement enabled the lawyers to characterize the brutishness in clinical terms, both figuratively and literally. Convincing Americans—even Bush administration lawyers—to openly allow torture would have been too hard a sell. The CIA's doctors enabled the agency to finesse this problem through artful definition.

This finesse also protected the doctors themselves. Numerous codes of medical ethics prohibit physician participation in torture. The most widely cited such code, passed by the United Nations General Assembly in December 1982, not only bars "participation" and "complicity" in torture; it also warns that "it is a contravention of medical ethics for health personnel . . . [t]o apply their knowledge and skills in order to assist in the interrogation of prisoners and detainees in a manner that may adversely affect the physical or mental health or condition of such prisoners or detainees *and which is not in accordance with the relevant international instruments.*"[74]

This language leaves plenty of space for parsing. It *permits* doctors to assist interrogators—even if what they do "may adversely affect the . . . health" of prisoners—so long as interrogation stays within the bounds of international law. And according to the Bush administration's lawyers, medical assistance itself was grounds for claiming that enhanced interrogation was compatible with international law.[75] The doctors' participation itself was thus reason for concluding that their participation was ethical—a tour de force of circular reasoning!

This ethical "reasoning" has ongoing legal bite. State medical licensing boards have the power to punish physicians for ethical lapses by suspending or revoking their licenses. People can sue doctors for harm caused by unethical conduct. And hospitals can refuse to grant admitting privileges to physicians with ethically dubious pasts. CIA doctors dread a storm surge of disciplinary complaints and lawsuits by human rights activists, former detainees, and others. And they fear that their pasts will haunt them, should they seek post-CIA careers as clinical caregivers. They've avoided these risks, so far, by staying anonymous—something the clandestine status of "enhanced" interrogation has enabled them to do. But keeping one's career under cover has its professional costs, and succeeding at doing so is hardly a sure thing. Being able to argue that they acted ethically, in the nation's service, thus matters greatly to these doctors. The legal architecture under which they served empowers them to do so.

That the clinical science supporting this legal architecture was questionable didn't concern the CIA. The agency's most senior officials deferred to the doctors, some of whom weren't shy about stretching the science. The CIA's disregard for science even extended to Mitchell's arguments for "enhanced" interrogation. Hubbard, who introduced Mitchell to counterterror policy makers and still insists that his methods worked, claims that Mitchell had good science behind him but that the agency's leadership didn't care. "The CIA is only interested in results," he told me. "Their eyes glaze over when you start talking science, research."

A Battle of Brawn

Disregard for the science was evident as the CIA scaled up its use of enhanced methods. The agency stuck to the Biderman-Seligman story, telling
administration lawyers that "the goal of interrogation is to create a state of
learned helplessness."[76] But a CIA background paper on enhanced interrogation reveals a descent into raw thuggishness. Instead of wearing away resistance through such measures as prolonged isolation and sleep deprivation,
black-site interrogators tried immediately to intimidate. Slaps to the face
and stomach, throwing detainees against a wall ("flexible," we're reassured),
and hosing with cold water became part of the mix within a day or two of a
detainee's arrival. Such acts pit the prisoner's will against the interrogator's.
They *provoke* anger, thereby *stiffening* resistance.

But they offer a heady payoff: the chance to go mano-a-mano with "the
worst of the worst" in a battle of brawn. A December 2004 CIA descrip-
tion of the "prototypical interrogation" is clinical in its tone but clear about
what black-site interrogators did. Within hours of "admission" to a secret
site, the detainee was stripped naked, shackled, and placed in a "walling collar." Interrogators then told their captive that they "will do what it takes to
get important information." They backed this up with slaps to the face and
stomach when the detainee did or said "anything inconsistent with the interrogators' instructions." And, said CIA officials, "once it becomes clear" that
the detainee "is lying, withholding information, or using other resistance
techniques," interrogators hurl him repeatedly against a wall—the "walling"
for which the collar was designed.[77] Whether this bullying yielded lifesaving
intelligence will long remain a matter of debate. What's indisputable is that
it channeled American outrage over the murder of 3,000 people on 9/11 and
the frightening sense of vulnerability that followed.

In its "Guidelines" for the black sites, the CIA's medical office said "enhanced" interrogation is "designed to psychologically 'dislocate' the detainee," to "maximize his feeling of vulnerability and helplessness." Dislocation
and vulnerability are what vast numbers of Americans felt in 9/11's wake.
"Enhanced" interrogation turned this feeling back onto those who attacked

us—or, at least, onto the few whom we'd managed to take alive. It brought some of us, therefore, security of the psychic sort—a sense, however chimerical, that we could assert control in the face of sudden, dislocating helplessness. And the doctors who supervised the black sites fed that sense of control, or its illusion, by lending an aura of precision and constraint to a ferocious endeavor.

Dr. Burney

Within the CIA's black-site archipelago, enhanced interrogation remained a cottage industry. The armed services, by contrast, embraced it on an industrial scale. By the early spring of 2002, Mitchell's and Jessen's proposal to mine SERE methods for actual interrogation had spread to every theater of post-9/11 warfare. It moved through chains of command, from JPRA to Joint Forces Command and the Pentagon, then to the regional commands responsible for Afghanistan and Guantanamo Bay. And it spread virally among lower-ranking officers who wondered how to get useful information from new captives.

At the highest levels of government, there was near certainty that men held at Guantanamo knew about plots in progress, secret cells, and the whereabouts of Al Qaeda leaders. Guantanamo's commander for intelligence gathering, Major General Michael Dunlavey, was under growing pressure to report breakthroughs. And the toughness of the Mitchell model fit his own take on the men he held, an impression influenced by his years as a juvenile court judge. He had lots of experience with kids who didn't feel guilt—teens who dealt drugs or did worse, without a sense of remorse. The detainees being offloaded from Afghanistan, he told me years later, weren't so different. "They're sociopaths," he said. "They like to kill. They use the excuse of religion to justify it."[78] And they'd respond to rewards and punishment.

In June 2002, a young psychiatrist, Major Paul Burney, and a clinical psychologist, Major John Leso, arrived at Guantanamo, expecting to treat soldiers with mental health problems.[79] So it came as a surprise to both that Dunlavey had assigned them to Guantanamo's new Behavioral Science Consultation Team, part of Joint Task Force 170, the unit responsible for interrogation. "[We] were hijacked," Dr. Burney recalled in 2007.[80] Like Scott Uithol when he landed in Baghdad, neither had any training or experience in interrogation. Burney was a general psychiatrist with some forensic experience; Leso had developed some expertise in the stresses associated with flight. When I spoke with Dunlavey, he acknowledged their lack of background but defended involving them anyway. "Nobody," he said, "knew what to do."

Dr. Burney, though, would become a central figure in the spread of interrogation methods bordering on torture to Guantanamo, then Abu Ghraib. In an e-mail interview, he acknowledged his role, but he insisted he'd voiced misgivings from the start, misgivings that his chain of command ignored. Who at Guantanamo made the ultimate decision to adopt SERE methods is likely to remain a mystery, shrouded in selective memory lapses and incompatible denials. But the basics are clear from interviews with participants in the decision, statements made to Senate Armed Services Committee investigators, and documents that have emerged from government inquiries.

For starters, Dunlavey had decided to "get rough," whether on his own initiative or under pressure from Washington. "There was pressure for immediate results," Burney told me, "frequent pressure to produce daily or . . . weekly 'breakthrough' of new intelligence information."[81] And there was, he said "pressure to find a link between Iraq and Al Qaeda" as the Bush administration built its case for war to remove Saddam from power.

Rumsfeld's List

It was in this charged context that Drs. Burney and Leso reached out to the army's chief SERE psychologist, Lieutenant Colonel Louie "Morgan" Banks, to arrange training in SERE techniques. "The psychologist on the team [Leso] personally knew Colonel Morgan Banks from prior experiences," Burney explained. "We thought that if there was any place in the army that could teach us about interrogation in general, it would be Colonel Banks and the army SERE school. Colonel Banks knew and we knew our supervisors wanted us to bring back a 'how-to' list of interrogation techniques."

Banks delivered. He arranged with JPRA for a September training session at Fort Bragg (home to the army SERE school), run by psychologist Gary Percival, who'd taught CIA interrogators two months earlier.[82] The four-day program included presentations on "rough handling," disruption of sleep cycles, "walling," exploitation of phobias, and exposure to cold.[83] Percival insisted to me in an interview that he had no idea how Burney and Leso might use the training (a claim undermined by the fact that four Guantanamo interrogators took part in the program[84]). Banks knew full well what Burney and Leso had in mind. But Banks convinced Burney that use of SERE techniques would backfire. "The goal of the SERE school," Burney told me, "is ultimately to bolster a soldier's ability to resist interrogations, and implementation of similar techniques with detainees would likely do the same."

Kirk Hubbard and James Mitchell wouldn't have disagreed. The SERE experience was designed to inoculate "captives" against learned helplessness; the Mitchell model meant to induce it. Journalists who've said that Mitchell reverse-engineered SERE[85] missed this point. Mitchell *reengineered* SERE to achieve what SERE trainers sought to guard against. Burney and Leso missed this distinction as well.[86] They left Fort Bragg with a list of harsh tactics but without an understanding of how to use them to do what Mitchell envisioned.

Despite his doubts, Dr. Burney pressed ahead. Within a few weeks of his return to Guantanamo, he'd drafted a memo with a list of SERE techniques. He told Senate Armed Services Committee investigators that there was "a lot of pressure to use more coercive techniques" and that if his memo didn't include them, "it wasn't going to go very far."[87] Burney's memo went far indeed. It went up his chain of command, to Dunlavey, then to Southern Command (which oversaw Guantanamo), and then to the Pentagon. There were some tweaks along the way. Simulated suffocation with a wet towel was added; a few items were subtracted, but Burney's list of "techniques" remained mostly intact. On December 2, Secretary of Defense Donald Rumsfeld approved the proposed "techniques," famously writing below his signature, "I stand for 8–10 hours a day. Why is standing limited to 4 hours?"[88]

Remarkably, Burney warned in his memo that his own proposals were dangerous and wouldn't work. SERE techniques, he'd written, put detainees' "physical and/or mental health" at risk and were "likely to garner inaccurate information and create an increased level of resistance."[89] But this caveat was edited out—"simply ignored and cut," he told me—before his proposal made its way off the island and farther up the chain of command.

Rumsfeld's sign-off formally applied only to Guantanamo but was widely taken as broader approval. Word spread to Afghanistan and, months later, to Iraq that the gloves were off—that it was okay, even desirable, to get tough with terrorists by tapping the list of methods Burney had devised. Local commanders varied the sequencing (and some of the techniques). But the SERE classics—slaps, stress positions, sleep deprivation, nudity, isolation, walling, and water-dousing—were almost always part of the repertoire. Dunlavey's successor, Major General Geoffrey Miller, not only embraced Burney's coercive scheme with ardor at Guantanamo; he brought the approach to Iraq when Pentagon officials sent him there a year later to "Gitmo-ize" interrogation. "You have to treat them like dogs," Miller reportedly said,[90] circling back, unwittingly or otherwise, to the new interrogation model's origins in Martin Seligman's studies of learned helplessness. The Abu Ghraib Biscuit on which Scott Uithol served was Miller's idea.

Looking Back

Dunlavey took advantage of Burney's standing as a psychiatrist to gain clinical legitimacy for a get-tough approach. Dr. Burney, though, was no mere cog in the machine. More than he preferred to admit after the fact, he took the initiative, consulting colleagues, then crafting a coercive plan. But he judged that the plan wouldn't work—a conclusion disregarded by superiors intent on their get-tough course. Like the CIA's leaders and the lawyers who immunized the Mitchell model, the chain of military command cared much less about the professional rationale for (or against) fierce tactics than about the feel-good message of precision and restraint that medical involvement sent.

As liberals who believe Burney and other military and CIA doctors should face professional discipline have warned, this feel-good message makes room for treatment of prisoners to become more dangerous. Surprisingly, perhaps, Burney agrees. "I think having a BSCT [Biscuit] gives interrogation practices an illusion of medical endorsement," he told me, "even if the BSCT team has no voice in actually approving or disapproving interrogation policies." The risk created is that the presence of doctors signals interrogators that they needn't worry about setting limits. The docs will keep things from going too far, or so the interrogators assume. Meanwhile, there's a pull on doctors to show that they're part of the team—to let interrogators push boundaries, especially when boundaries are blurry. The net effect of this dialog of expectations, as Jonathan Marks has suggested,[91] may be to let the ferocity go further than it otherwise might.

Yet Dr. Burney turns this argument back on itself. By contributing to interrogation policy and practice at Guantanamo, he believed, he could set limits: "People have written that I should have simply not participated at all. In retrospect, perhaps that would have [been] best for my own self interest, but I had been educated about the Zimbardo effect, and I knew what would happen if a group of interrogators was simply left alone with a group of detainees with no directions or boundaries for a long enough period of time."

What *can* happen—what *did* happen at Abu Ghraib, Burney argues—is descent into sadism. In psychologist Philip Zimbardo's mock prison, set in a Stanford basement, nine "guards," responsible for nine "prisoners" (all student volunteers randomly assigned to their roles) and left unsupervised, became shockingly abusive over just a few days.[92] Guantanamo interrogators, Burney said, "were woefully underprepared." Biscuit doctors could draw on their clinical experience to offer guidance and impose restraint. But, he said, "seasoned, experienced interrogators would have been a much better option than us."

Dr. Burney's situational defense of the ethics of his Biscuit service is at odds with the argument the Pentagon made—that medical ethics were beside the point because Biscuit doctors didn't act as physicians. "I tried my best," he told me, "not to be a doc when I was at [Guantanamo]. I had my

Geneva Convention card changed from noncombatant to combatant status. I refused to medically evaluate or treat detainees. Try as I might though, I can't help it. I am a doc."

Could Dr. Burney have refused Biscuit service—or, at least, declined to draft the list of techniques that Rumsfeld eventually approved? Typically, army physicians can raise ethical concerns with senior colleagues via the military's distinctive, medical chain of command. Within the armed forces, medicine maintains a surprising degree of autonomy. Doctors serve in separate, clinical units with distinctive legal protections and obligations. They're noncombatants under international law (even army cooks are considered combatants; clergy are the only others with similar standing). Opposing forces can't attack them, and they're not permitted to fight: They can carry arms but they're allowed to use them only in self-defense. They're expected—under army regulations and international law—to adhere to established precepts of medical ethics. And they're required by the Geneva Conventions, the main source of the law of war, to treat friend and foe alike, prioritizing care based on clinical need.

Biscuit service was a radical departure. Biscuit doctors were deployed as combatants, apart from medical units. "A [Biscuit] team," Burney observed, "is the only place I've ever heard of in the army where the doc's chain of command is completely out of the medical system." Dr. Burney reported to a combatant commander. He had no *medical* superior with whom to raise his concerns about the ethics of his role. Moreover, a military intelligence officer (the colonel who supervised him) and Generals Dunlavey and Miller were responsible for his performance evaluations. To do other than comply with their orders posed an enormous career risk. It could even have gotten him court-martialed. Military law requires obedience to commands unless they're "patently illegal."[93]

Burney could have argued before a court-martial that what he'd been asked to do was illegal, both because the harsh tactics violated military law and because medical complicity in such abuse was unethical. Military regulations require medical officers to adhere to professional ethics, which, in turn, proscribe complicity in tactics contrary to international law. But Dunlavey had obtained a legal memo from Guantanamo's Judge Advocate General officer approving the techniques.[94] This was enough to establish that they weren't *patently* unlawful—and that medical assistance in designing and employing them was, therefore, not *patently* unethical. Had Burney refused to prepare the proposed list of coercive techniques, he could have been court-martialed and convicted.

Discussion of the awkward fit between Biscuit service and Hippocratic ideals was, in short, silenced by career anxieties, legal apprehension, and the command scheme at Guantanamo. The claim that Biscuit doctors didn't act as clinicians and that medical ethics thus didn't apply substituted for serious conversation about ethics. Secrecy protected Biscuit doctors and their commanders from accountability for this arrangement until the midnight wilding at Abu Ghraib led to exposure of the interrogation policy that Burney helped to fashion.

chapter eight

doctors as warriors II

ethics and politics

Had the doctors who planned or oversaw national security interrogation in 9/11's wake turned to their professional societies for ethical guidance, they'd have found none. To be sure, there were platitudes about not participating in torture, but there wasn't anything resembling clarity about how "torture" should be defined. Nor did these groups draw lines between acceptable and impermissible participation in interrogation or other warfighting activities short of torture. This left them at a loss when, despite the Bush administration's best efforts at secrecy, it became public that military physicians and psychologists had played roles in post-9/11 interrogation.

The disconnect between Americans' sense of basic decency and the ferocity authorized at high levels of government made an unraveling of the secrecy inevitable. Abu Ghraib, though, was the catalyst. The photos begged questions and begat inquiries. Released documents dropped hints. Dismayed military officers leaked details. Scholars and journalists began the years-long effort to assemble the larger picture. With my colleague Jonathan Marks, I joined in this effort. On January 6, 2005, we published an article in the *New England Journal of Medicine* that set off a firestorm—in the media and among health professionals. We reported for the first time, based on interviews with military sources as well as documents made public through the Freedom of Information Act (FOIA), that "behavioral science consultation teams" advised interrogators on the use of harsh tactics at Abu Ghraib and Guantanamo.[1] We knew nothing at that point about the adoption of SERE (survival, evasion, resistance, and escape) methods, but we'd learned that psychologists and psychiatrists served on these teams and used medical records to help plan interrogations.

Outraged editorial writers, human rights advocates, physicians, psychologists, and others condemned the participating doctors for violating their Hippocratic commitment to patient well-being. Most dismissed the Pentagon's defense—that the doctor who assists interrogators doesn't "function . . . as a physician" and needn't heed Hippocratic ideals.[2] But they offered little by way of explanation for their objections to involvement in interrogation, coercive or otherwise. Was complicity in torture—or other conduct that violated the laws of war—the only problem? Or was participation in all interrogation objectionable, since it didn't yield benefits for "patients" and might, in fact, do people harm? How should "torture" and "participation" be defined? And if involvement in interrogation was problematic per se, how might this be squared with medicine's myriad public roles, including clinical evaluation and courtroom testimony bearing on criminal defendants' culpability?

That professional associations hadn't spoken to these questions troubled those who feared that military doctors were running amok. It also unnerved psychologists, psychiatrists, and other clinicians who'd participated in the development of harsh interrogation strategies or overseen actual interrogations. They feared professional discipline, criminal prosecution, and lasting damage to their reputations. Silence from their professional associations meant that their actions weren't specifically proscribed. But it allowed their critics to invoke amorphous language—prohibitions against participating in torture or doing harm—as a basis for judging them.

"A Tool of Appeasement?"

It was in this charged context that I received a call from the ethics director of the American Psychological Association (APA), Steve Behnke, a few days after our January 2005 *New England Journal of Medicine* article came out.

He'd known me in law school, seen our piece, and wanted to meet for lunch. Over cheap PanAsian, he pressed me on what I knew about what military psychologists had done. After Yale Law School, he'd taken an atypical turn, passing on law firm pay to pursue a Ph.D. in clinical psychology. But he'd made his way back to the realm of ethics and law, taking charge of the ethics office at the APA less than a year before the 9/11 attacks.

Along the way, he'd impressed successive supervisors with his smarts, willingness to listen, and ability to anticipate their needs. That's what he was trying to do, with no small difficulty, when we got together. Many APA members had reacted to the *New England Journal* piece by demanding investigations and condemnation of Biscuit psychologists. Journalists and human rights groups were asking questions and watching closely. Meanwhile, out of public view, psychologists who saw the War on Terror as a historic growth opportunity for the profession were pressing for a permissive approach to the ethics of service on behalf of the nation's security. Within the APA, these psychologists held sway. The association's president, his successor, and the group's lobbying arm were intent on controlling damage to the APA's relations with the military. Members' Pentagon contracts and grants worth tens of millions were at stake, along with their patriotic feelings. So were the careers of military psychologists who'd taught and planned fierce interrogations.

Behnke asked me what I'd do if I were him. I said I didn't know. He gently suggested there wasn't proof that military psychologists had done anything wrong. I agreed that there wasn't nearly enough proof to punish anyone, but, I said, there was more than enough to ask undiplomatic questions. The public and the profession needed to know more about what doctors had been asked to do, had already done, and might be called on to do in the future. And the country needed to know the larger context: the origins of interrogation practices bordering on torture and the reasons for involvement by psychologists, physicians, and other health professionals. Professional associations, I realized, couldn't conduct such an inquiry— they had neither subpoena power nor security clearances. But they could, I said, call for one, by Congress or an independent commission. Blind

deference to the administration's denials, justifications, and claims of secrecy would sacrifice a central tenet of professionalism: independent say on
questions of right conduct affecting a profession's relationships to clients
and society.[3]

I urged Behnke to reject the Pentagon's proposition that doctors who
plan or oversee interrogation needn't heed clinical ethics. And I implored
him to reject the torture memo writers' efforts to define America's obligations downward so as to permit practices condemned by international law.
Deferring to the torture memos, I pointed out, would make the ethical prohibition against participating in torture meaningless in practice. It would
give health professionals involved in abusive interrogation a free pass. And
it would put professionals who said "no" at greater risk for military prosecution, since they'd be hard-pressed to make the case that participation in practices sanctioned by their professional societies is unethical and thus "patently
illegal." Behnke assured me that the APA would speak clearly on both fronts,
affirming that clinical ethics applied to psychologists who used clinical skills
to aid interrogators and that international law's definition of "torture" would
be the group's ethical anchor.

A month later, the APA's president named a ten-person "task force" on
national security interrogation. Six members were military psychologists; five
had taught, advised, or overseen interrogators at Guantanamo, Abu Ghraib,
bases in Afghanistan, or clandestine sites elsewhere. One was Morgan Banks,
who'd arranged training in SERE methods for Guantanamo interrogation
teams at Paul Burney's request, then gone on to write rules for Biscuit doctors at Guantanamo and elsewhere. Another was Scott Shumate, who'd battled over turf with Kirk Hubbard and Jim Mitchell inside the Central Intelligence Agency's Counter-Terrorism Center, then joined Mitchell on his flight
to Bangkok to interrogate Abu Zubaydah. Shumate had since left the CIA
for a Pentagon position as chief psychologist for counter-terror programs,
responsible for (among other matters) threat assessment of Guantanamo detainees.[4] A third was Larry James, who'd taken over the Guantanamo Biscuit
when Burney and John Leso rotated out, then, on Banks's recommendation,
succeeded Scott Uithol at Abu Ghraib. Another SERE psychologist, Bryce

Lefever, had advised interrogators in Afghanistan and was sympathetic to the Mitchell-Jessen approach.

Given these conflicts of interest, the report of the task force was hardly a surprise. Not only did the panel endorse interrogation as a new "area of practice" for psychologists; it embraced the Bush administration's claim that doctors who work in this field needn't concern themselves with clinical ethics. All they need do to loosen themselves from Hippocratic obligation is to tell their prisoners that they aren't acting as therapists. "Psychologists," the report said, "have a special responsibility to clarify their role in situations where individuals may have an incorrect impression that psychologists are serving in a health care provider role."[5] Disclosure, even without consent, dissolves the ethical problem, or so the authors claimed. Even breaches of clinical confidentiality are okay (Biscuit doctors had access to prisoners' medical records), the report said, so long as "[p]sychologists take care not to leave a misimpression that information is confidential when in fact it is not." The only "ethical obligation" psychologists have to "individuals who are not their clients" (read "detainees") is to "ensure that their activities . . . are safe, legal, and ethical." This was circularity without shame.

More stunning was the panel's rejection of international law in favor of the Bush administration's bid to redefine torture. The task force did so in disguised fashion, using language that at once reassured casual readers and delivered immunity from professional discipline to psychologists who conceived and oversaw SERE-based interrogation. "Psychologists do not engage in behaviors that violate the laws of the United States," the panel's report stated.[6] But then came the small print. "Psychologists involved in national security-related activities," the report said, "follow all applicable rules and regulations that govern their roles. Over the course of the recent United States military presence in locations such as Afghanistan, Iraq, and Cuba [Guantanamo], such rules and regulations have been significantly developed and refined."[7]

What had been "significantly developed and refined" were the torture memos, which gave a pass to the gamut of SERE-based interrogation strategies—and to the psychologists and psychiatrists who fashioned and oversaw them. Military psychologists, according to the task force, had a *duty* to participate in such interrogations if ordered to do so, since these orders were both legal and ethical. Instead of supporting mental health professionals who, out of conscience, disobey, the panel helped to criminalize noncompliance, since soldiers must, by law, follow orders unless they are "patently illegal."

For casual readers, the task force suggested otherwise, stating that "[a]n ethical reason for psychologists to not follow the law is to act 'in keeping with basic principles of human rights.'" For military officers, though, this language offered no protection from career-ending rebuke and criminal sanction. That's because the panel didn't *require* psychologists to refuse, on ethical grounds, to "follow the law." To the contrary, the task force said that if psychologists cannot resolve "conflicts between ethics and law," they "*may* adhere to the requirements of the law" (emphasis added). "Ethics" were voluntary. But in the military, lawful orders are mandatory, leaving psychologists with no basis for refusing to participate.[8]

The task force met just once, for two days in June 2005. On the eve of the meeting, as the group gathered for dinner, Steve Behnke learned of a development he knew wouldn't please the military participants. The lead story in the next day's *New York Times,* just released online, would report that psychologists and psychiatrists at Guantanamo "aided interrogators in conducting and refining coercive interrogations of detainees" and gave "advice on how to increase stress levels and exploit fears." The piece, by Neil Lewis, was based on interviews he'd done with former interrogators and on an article by Jonathan Marks and me, released hours before by the *New England Journal of Medicine.* The two articles offered the first, sketchy account of Guantanamo's Behavioral Science Consultation Team, including its custom-tailoring of stressors to break detainees' resistance and its use of prisoners' medical information to plan interrogations.

Later inquiries by Senate investigators, journalists, and scholars would confirm these accounts[9] and lay out the Guantanamo story in greater detail. But when Behnke arrived at the restaurant with printouts of the two pieces, he met fierce denial. "I remember being at dinner the night before and Steve coming in," an attendee later told me. "He had a copy of your paper and also a copy of the newspaper article. It evoked quite a strong reaction." The articles were "false," full of "lies," several of the military psychologists insisted. The presence of psychologists, they maintained, had saved lives—indeed, Scott Shumate claimed to have personally done so. Larry James, who'd run Biscuits at both Abu Ghraib and Guantanamo, said psychologists "can be whistleblowers," the dinner attendee recalled. James, he said, "argued very strongly that if you pull psychologists out of those situations, people will die."

Marks and I were scheduled to speak to the group the next day, at Behnke's invitation, about the ethical challenges posed by military doctors' conflicting roles. At the dinner, this idea didn't go over well. "Scott Shumate," a participant recalled, "argued very forcefully that to give an open forum to people who are openly telling lies would destroy the credibility . . . of what we were trying to do. . . . Those feelings were so vehement that Steve basically took the reins and said that step, of inviting [us] into the meeting, was not going to be productive or appropriate."

So we were disinvited, and the next morning, a Friday, the panel reassembled in a surly mood. After agreeing on boilerplate language condemning complicity in torture, the group turned to its real tasks: settling on how to define torture and whether to sanction interrogation as a legitimate area of practice. (The panel voted to keep its discussions confidential, but interviews with members, on condition of anonymity, made it possible to learn the gist.) Military members pushed for ethical and legal cover, fretting that fallout from reports like Lewis's and ours could lead to career-ending censure and worse. Banks, James, Shumate, and others said psychologists hadn't harmed detainees and that the armed forces' internal investigative procedures sufficed. Behnke lent them critical support, insisting that claims of abuse were unfounded.[10] They easily won over their civilian colleagues. "People . . . said, look, psychologists are good guys, and you don't want them to be prosecuted," recalled one member.

By Saturday, when the meeting adjourned, its military participants had prevailed. Within a week, the panel's report became APA policy, approved by the association's board on an "emergency" basis.[11] On a confidential listserv, used by group members to air views, the chair was explicit about the report's deference to the administration's permissive policy:

> [W]e should keep two points in mind. First, we discussed the role of human rights standards for the document, and it seems that our colleagues from the military were clear that including such standards in the document would likely (perhaps definitely) put the document at odds with United States law and military regulations. The effect of such a conflict, it seems to me, would be that the military would simply have ignored the document—thus, the community that we would most want to reach would have been prevented from using the report.[12]

When, a few weeks after the APA adopted the report, the *New York Times* reported that top military lawyers had risked their careers by insisting that human rights law governed and that participants in harsh interrogation could be prosecuted, three of the panel's four nonmilitary members developed buyer's remorse. Nina Thomas, a psychoanalyst and student of war trauma who'd earlier gone along with the group's rejection of international human rights principles (and called the report "beyond impressive"), told fellow task force members: "I can't continue to read the popular press and feel sanguine about our work." "I am hopeful," she added, "that Rumsfeld might be arrested."[13] Meanwhile, Pentagon officials made the report part of their Biscuit "standard operating procedure." They referred to it repeatedly as they pushed back against charges that they'd enlisted doctors to plan torture.

By midsummer, bloggers, editorialists, and activists were condemning the APA for countenancing human rights abuse and violations of the laws of war. Amid this growing criticism, the panel's discussions devolved into fratricide. Two more nonmilitary members chastised the APA and the task force for refusing to define torture by reference to human rights law. One, Jean Maria Arrigo, called the task force "a tool of appeasement." The other quit in protest. APA president Gerald Koocher wasn't shy about striking back. "I have zero interest," he said on the listserv, "in entangling APA with the nebulous, toothless, contradictory, and obfuscatory treaties that comprise 'international law.'"[14] When Arrigo charged on a radio talk show that APA leaders stacked the panel's membership and manipulated its procedures to ensure a good outcome for the Bush administration, Koocher wrote, in an "open letter" to the host, that Arrigo's dissenting views were due to her "history of personal trauma" and "underscored the sad emotional aftermath of a troubled upbringing."[15]

Over the next several years, the APA reversed most of the positions the task force had taken. Thousands of members demanded that it do so, embarrassed by fresh disclosures about the scope of psychologists' involvement in detainee abuse. Petition drives, referenda, and rising anger over the Pentagon's influence on the association forced the issue. The APA embraced international law's stricter approach to defining torture, forbade psychologists from consulting with interrogators in settings that violate international law, and in 2010 changed its ethics code to make respect for "human rights" mandatory, even if at odds with national "law, regulations, or other governing legal authority." But the psychologists who pioneered SERE-based interrogation years before could rest assured that the task force report still shielded them from career-threatening disciplinary sanctions. The report still stands as a statement of the rules that governed at the time.

It's easy to chide the APA for its interrogation ethics fiasco. But the larger disappointment was the APA's failure at every stage to face the question of whether and how to weigh Hippocratic benevolence against one or another vision of the social good. To his credit, Colonel Bryce Lefever pressed the task force to address it. Lefever, the son of a Protestant theologian who morphed from World War II conscientious objector to controversial Reagan appointee and human rights doubter,[16] argued that professional ethics should be about the common good. So long as roles are kept separate—so long as doctors who treat the enemy don't, at the same time, fight them—"do no harm" ought to mean protecting the community, he contended, whether as therapists or as warriors. There are, of course, other understandings of the relation between Hippocratic benevolence and social good—understandings that animate the bitter differences over doctors' work with interrogators. But rival understandings weren't clarified, and debate about them wasn't joined—neither in the task force discussions nor in the nasty public exchanges that followed. Claims that doctors should serve the social good by acting to keep America safe were countered with condemnations of any departure from Hippocratic benevolence.

A central theme of this book is that doctors routinely play non-Hippocratic roles. Koocher pressed this point to a fault, defending coercive interrogation on the ground that "[p]sychologists often do things that 'harm' one person for an appropriate societal purpose" and that much of this work is "coercive or less than fully voluntary"[17] (he pointed to assessments done for the law's purposes[18]). One needn't accept his parallel between coercion at Guantanamo and the county courthouse to take his point about the inevitability of non-Hippocratic roles. To dismiss them all merely drives them underground, a recipe for ethical discontrol. Such discontrol was evident when James Mitchell revisited Harold Wolff's and Albert Biderman's work, reformulated SERE, then made his case to CIA officials. And it was manifest when Paul Burney and John Leso reached out to Morgan Banks, then drew up a list of methods that the International Committee of the Red Cross would call "tantamount to torture."

"Kind of Brilliant in a Way"

The American Psychiatric Association took a less tolerant approach to interrogation—or so it seemed. In May 2006, the group announced a flat-out ban on its members' involvement—a ban not limited to torture. It proscribed all "direct participation," including "being present in the interrogation room, asking or suggesting questions, or advising authorities on the use of specific techniques of interrogation with particular detainees."[19] And it barred disclosure of medical records or "information derived from the treatment relationship" to interrogators. But it gave psychiatrists carte blanche to provide "training" on "areas within their professional expertise."[20] The idea was to keep psychiatrists from assessing individual detainees for interrogation purposes while allowing them to give more general advice.

On its face, this policy broke sharply with that of the American Psychological Association, which permitted its members to craft interrogation plans, suggest counterresistance strategies, and even question detainees. But more was less: The psychiatry APA issued its policy as a "Position Statement," which, under the organization's rules, isn't enforceable through disciplinary sanctions. The group's president at the time, Dr. Steven Sharfstein, admitted as much, noting that the Statement wasn't "an ethical rule" and assuring military psychiatrists that they "wouldn't get in trouble with the APA" for following orders that violate it.[21] Psychiatrists in the armed services got the message. A high-ranking army psychiatrist who spoke with me on condition of anonymity called it "kind of brilliant in a way." "Come out in a position statement so it looked in public like they're against it," he said. "It allows them to maintain the sanctity of the doctor-patient relationship . . . and appease the far-left people who don't distinguish between interrogation and torture." Meanwhile, he said, the statement gave psychiatrists a pass for their Biscuit service, since it didn't impose an enforceable duty to say no.

This psychiatrist served on a Biscuit for six months, after the APA issued its "Position Statement." In defiance of the "Statement," he and others watched interrogations,[22] offered feedback on interviewing technique, assessed detainees' resistance, and suggested ways to overcome it. "If it had been an ethical statement,"[23] he told me, "I would have never come near it [Biscuit service]."

Thus, in different ways, the professional groups representing psychologists and psychiatrists pushed participation in interrogation into a don't-ask-don't-tell netherworld. The psychology APA at first gave Biscuit members quiet carte blanche, ignoring the problem of harm to individuals without explaining why. When members rebelled against Pentagon influence, "do no harm" made an indiscriminate appearance, as a cudgel for condemning *all* activities that inflict harm for state or social purposes. This merely drove Biscuit psychologists underground—in some cases, literally into hiding—as APA members and others filed disciplinary charges against them. And when, after much acrimony, the APA settled on a solution, permitting participation within human rights law's constraints, it ignored the broader question of when clinical caregivers should and shouldn't compromise Hippocratic benevolence for public purposes.

The psychiatry APA's evasion of this broader question was more egregious. The association appeared to give a restrictive answer, barring assessment of "particular detainees" for interrogation purposes. But the association's "Position Statement" was little more than a ruse[24]—a way to quiet critics while allowing Biscuit psychiatrists safe harbor. For Biscuit psychiatrists, this deception came at a cost: the knowledge that their work was officially scorned by their peers. They could try to keep their Biscuit service a secret, but disrepute for doing one's duty is hardly a recipe for high morale. Nor is it a helpful military recruiting tool—or a career enhancer for doctors who leave the service to seek jobs in civilian life. Beyond this, the psychiatric association's failure to either bar Biscuit service or concede its legitimacy leaves military practitioners without their own professional body to turn to when questions arise about the contours of the Biscuit role. By clinging to the Hippocratic Myth for the sake of appearances, the association shut down discussion of the extent to which national security should trump the promise of fidelity to individuals. The ironic result was less protection for Hippocratic fidelity and benevolence than might have ensued from open consideration of the balance between these ideals and America's security.

Toward an Ethical Accommodation?

How should open consideration of this balance play out? For starters, consider the simple solution urged by the Pentagon in 2004, when word leaked out that doctors were helping to plan interrogations. Physicians who do so, the assistant secretary of defense for health affairs asserted, don't act as doctors and thus aren't bound by patient-oriented ethics. In an interview at the time, Dr. David Tornberg, deputy assistant secretary of defense for health affairs, drew an analogy to a physician who becomes a fighter pilot. "He's not functioning as a physician," Tornberg told me. He has no doctor-patient relationship with those at whom he takes aim. He can kill them, so long as he complies with the laws of war and the orders issued by his chain of command. His medical degree isn't a pledge of pacifism.

Tornberg was surely right about his fighter pilot, who neither uses his medical skills nor forges clinical relationships with his human targets. Doctors do a great deal without the burden of Hippocratic expectations. They run businesses and hold political office. We don't see a senator who advocates a troop surge in Afghanistan as a medical ethics offender because he's also an obstetrician; nor would we hold a heart surgeon who becomes president and orders an air strike accountable for breaching the Hippocratic Oath.

When, in the 1990s, psychiatrist Radovan Karadzic became leader of the Bosnian Serbs and orchestrated the murder of tens of thousands of Muslims, some saw irony in his professional past, but it didn't add to the war crimes charges against him. To be sure, doctors who've done heinous things beyond the bedside or clinic have faced professional sanctions. Murder, rape, and running guns to terrorists have been cause for discipline because doctors, like other professionals, are expected to maintain high moral character.[25] It's inconceivable that Karadzic, were he somehow to be freed from the prison at The Hague where he now resides, would be permitted by a licensing board to practice medicine. Yet Tornberg's point applies. Karadzic didn't act as a doctor. He didn't use clinical judgment or medical methods to kill or to inspire others to do so.

But the physicians and psychologists who planned and oversaw interrogation on the armed services' and the CIA's behalf did use their professional skills and judgment. James Mitchell, the master-designer of the SERE-based strategy, drew creatively on his clinical experience and command of theory. He made plausible inferences—more plausible than can be admitted in polite company—from available data on people's responses to stress. Paul Burney also relied on his clinical background, which gave him "street cred" with SERE psychologists and senior commanders as he developed the list that Rumsfeld blessed. And scores of "behavioral science consultants" since Burney have used their clinical judgment to assess detainees' coping styles and to spot vulnerabilities. Likewise, the CIA physicians who crafted protocols for waterboarding, walling, cold-water dousing, and the like to make them "medically appropriate" drew on both their clinical training and their readings of the medical literature.

No less important was the aura of benevolence and restraint that these professionals lent to interrogation through their caregiving credentials. Their presence reassured military leaders, CIA officials, and the torture memos' authors *because* of their "physicianhood" (I use this expression broadly, to encompass clinical psychology). Their identity as clinical caregivers signaled safety and legitimacy because of people's Hippocratic expectations. To claim that doctors who aid interrogators don't act as doctors is to take no notice of the technical skills, clinical judgment, and moral authority they bring to the intelligence-gathering mission.

Does this mean that doctors should eschew all involvement in interrogation—and all participation in their country's defense more generally? In the wake of the Abu Ghraib scandal, some medical ethics commentators and human rights activists urged this view, insisting that military and CIA clinicians should limit themselves to caregiving activities consonant with Hippocratic ideals.[26] But this appeal to purity misreads the concern that animates the Oath's promise of fidelity. Physicians since Hippocratic times have pledged their loyalty to patients as part of a win-win proposition: Inspire patients' trust and thereby gain their confidence—in doctors' explanations, nostrums, and words of reassurance. Patients "win" through the therapeutic benefits this confidence delivers[27]; doctors gain economic and social status from heightened desire for their services.[28] Fidelity and benevolence in clinical relations are at the core of this transaction. The Oath's key phrase—"into every house where I come, I will enter only for the good of my patients"—is a promise about the contours of a personal relationship.

Beyond the realm of one-to-one clinical relationships, the Oath's promise of fidelity and benevolence is less apropos. Use of biomedical science for social purposes absent a personal bond between doctor and clinical subject doesn't risk one-to-one betrayal of the sort that the Oath was meant to guard against. Government regulators routinely use medical knowledge to balance risks against benefits when assessing environmental and occupational hazards. Intelligence agencies have long employed psychological "profiles" of international leaders—from menaces like Mahmoud Ahmadinejad of Iran to more benign figures with whom America does diplomatic business. Psychiatrists and psychologists prepare these profiles, but they don't perform one-to-one clinical assessments; their raw material comes from public and classified sources.[29] To read the Oath as a commitment to use medical knowledge only for patient care is to demand a cultish purity that abjures the common good.

Thus war-fighting and other national security endeavors that enlist a doctor's knowledge sans a clinical relationship don't compromise the Hippocratic promise of fidelity and benevolence. Using drugs as weapons, for example—say, firing pharmaceutically-loaded shells at enemy troops or menacing crowds—can't fairly be condemned as a Hippocratic breach of faith. Such weaponry would raise a host of law-of-war issues: the Chemical Weapons Convention[30] draws a hazy distinction between use of chemicals to control crowds (legitimate) and to engage foreign or insurgent forces (unlawful). But whether the weapons designers are doctors or hold some other credential wouldn't matter to the analysis.

The question of drugs as weapons isn't an abstraction. The U.S. military and those of other countries have shown increasing interest in pharmaceutical approaches to calming crowds, subduing terrorists, and waging war. The Pentagon has explored weaponization of a variety of psychoactive drugs, including benzodiazepines (e.g., Valium), opiates, and other agents that influence alertness or mood.[31] Russia has gone further, employing fentanyl, a synthetic opiate, to end a 2002 standoff between security forces and Chechen terrorists who seized 800 hostages at a Moscow theater. (The results were disastrous; more than 100 hostages died.)

The risk of confusion over the role of Hippocratic ethics outside the clinical context was illustrated in 2007 by a British Medical Association (BMA) report on drugs as weapons.[32] The report concluded that "doctors should not knowingly use their skills and knowledge for weapons development" because "the duty to avoid doing harm rises above . . . a duty to contribute to national security." Were weapons development something that doctors did within the scope of clinical relationships, this conclusion would make sense, as an adjunct to Hippocratic priority for the well-being of clinical subjects.

But the BMA didn't claim to find a clinical tie between weapons developers and those in the crosshairs. The BMA's asserted "duty to avoid doing harm" is a duty to society more generally, not merely to clinical subjects. It's well-meaning sentiment. As ethics, though, it's imperial overreach. Hippocratic ethics is an ethics of professional role, critical to clinical relationships but not a general guide for public policy. Physicians can and should speak to national security matters as citizens, but it's a category mistake for them to apply clinical ethics to policy matters beyond the reach of their clinical role.

Doing so, moreover, adds little. A general "duty to avoid doing harm" provides no policy guidance. It's virtually content-free. So the BMA's announcement that duty to avoid harm "rises above" duty to contribute to national security lacks meaning. These two "duties" are faces of the same ill-defined goal. The question of how best to secure a nation against harm is a matter of policy, not clinical ethics. Doctors, no more or less than anyone else, have a *legal* duty to abide by the rules of war (including the Chemical Weapons Convention). They shouldn't invoke clinical ethics to answer policy questions that don't involve clinical relationships.

Teaching interrogators good interview technique is of a piece with other forms of public service that don't involve a bond between doctor and clinical subject. Coaching interrogators on how to foster a relationship—how to look for common ground, connect viscerally, and nurture a sense of reciprocal obligation—doesn't demand that the *doctor* form a bond with detainees. The doctor can keep to a classroom role or offer individualized guidance, by viewing videotaped interrogations and suggesting strategies. So long as the doctor's involvement isn't known to those being interrogated, there's no professional relationship and thus no risk of Hippocratic betrayal. The doctor can still do wrong—by countenancing tactics that violate human rights or the laws of war—but this isn't *Hippocratic* wrongdoing.

Making a personal appearance is another matter. The clinician who joins in the questioning or who performs face-to-face assessments for interrogation purposes establishes a professional relationship, with its unspoken premise of Hippocratic fidelity and benevolence. Scott Uithol's disclaimer, "I'm not your doctor," borrowed from the practice of forensic psychiatry, isn't enough to make this premise go away. I say more about this in the next chapter, when I consider medicine's expanding role in the courtroom. Here I limit myself to pointing out that people's expectations of medicine—expectations that are viscerally felt, culturally embedded, and imbued since childhood—aren't amenable to easy reset, based on a single act of disclosure. Once the doctor becomes an interrogator, Hippocratic betrayal is part of the picture.

The psychiatry APA missed this distinction. Its "Position Statement" on interrogation puts "suggesting questions" and "advising authorities on the use of specific techniques" with "particular detainees" off limits, whether or not psychiatrists make personal contact with prisoners. But the "Statement" allows psychiatrists to question prisoners and offer opinions to courts and correctional authorities—if prisoners are awaiting trial or serving time. The "Statement," that is, treats the practice of forensic psychiatry more permissively, even though the outcome of an adverse forensic evaluation can be catastrophic.[33] Criminal conviction, a life spent in prison, a sentence of death—these are among the potential consequences of making a bad impression on a doctor empowered to opine in court. Surely, a clinical assessment that makes such consequences more likely is as much a betrayal of Hippocratic expectations as is advice to military interrogators about how to exploit a detainee's vulnerabilities.

Does this mean that doctors should decline per se to form relationships with clinical subjects (an awkward term, but we're not talking about patients here) for national security or criminal justice reasons? Hippocratic purists say yes, noting that these public reasons are at odds with medicine's caregiving role. If chided for being unconcerned about the common good, they're inclined to reply that professionals—including doctors and lawyers—best serve the public interest through undiluted commitment to their clients' well-being. But this faith-based proposition leaves no room for the possibility that doctors can contribute more directly to the common good, a possibility that's growing as biomedical science advances.

I consider medicine's potential contributions to criminal and civil justice in the next chapter; here I note some possibilities on the national security front. Psychiatric assessments are a Cold War–era standby, used to vet clandestine informants, spies and counterspies, and the like. But medical technologies that seem the stuff of sci-fi are coming online. Brain imaging, especially functional magnetic resonance imaging, which tracks metabolic activity throughout the brain (by measuring blood oxygen levels), is generating excitement beyond its confirmed capabilities.[34] The hope is that neurologists will be able to tie patterns of brain activity to truth-telling and thereby ferret out lies.[35] Startup firms are already marketing this and other imaging technologies to the intelligence community,[36] and there are accounts of its having been tried in combat theaters on a small scale.

Potential uses of mind-altering drugs are also multiplying. The pharmacology of the 1963 Kubark manual, which called for giving drugs to daze and confuse, is crude by comparison to current possibilities. A decade ago, the army's SERE school invited Yale psychiatrist Andrew Morgan to study the biochemistry of hopelessness and resilience during resistance training. Over the next seven years, Morgan and others took blood samples from trainees at multiple stages of their "captivity," looking for chemical markers of states of mind. What they found enabled them to glimpse the outlines of a stress management system that typically sustains our resilience but that can collapse under the weight of extreme experience. Blood testosterone levels remain stable, or even rise, when men under stress become, as Dr. Morgan put it to me in an interview, "invigorated and mad." But these levels plunge when anxiety and fear send men into "flight mode."[37]

Serum levels of a protein known as neuropeptide Y offered another look at resilience. When stress makes us "invigorated and mad," our neuroendocrine systems ramp up release of norepinephrine, mobilizing our minds, muscles, and energy reserves for action. Norepinephrine, though, has a downside. It empowers us to act, but it wears down body and spirit. Too much norepinephrine pushes our anxiety above optimal levels, toward the breakdown of confidence and means-ends thinking that Martin Seligman called learned helplessness. Neuropeptide Y limits this down side. It enables us to use norepinephrine more efficiently (so we need less), and it inhibits norepinephrine release. SERE trainees who kept up high neuropeptide Y concentrations during abuse were more resilient and less likely to show signs of learned helplessness. They were better at dodging and weaving in response to their "interrogators'" questions. They remained clear-headed, resisted their captors, and received high performance ratings from their instructors. Conversely, trainees with lower neuropeptide Y levels were more wont to become confused and depressed. Like students who "choke" on a big test, their performance crashed.

These and other findings make it possible to tailor resistance training to each soldier's neurobiological strengths and weaknesses. More than that, they open the way to drug treatment to boost resilience and temper the symptoms of posttraumatic stress disorder. But they also offer *actual* interrogators a new way to track the progress of their efforts to "break" prisoners—by monitoring chemical markers of confusion and despair. Beyond this, our emerging understanding of the physiology of stress management raises the sci-fi scenario of chemical intervention to *block* the biological feedback loops that support resilience. Drug "treatment" could *induce* learned helplessness—and confusion and despair. Advances in the neurobiology of stress are open to dual use: They empower doctors to bolster human resilience—and to go rogue by breaking it down.

And consider a few pharmacological possibilities, perhaps farther over the horizon, for our own fighting men and women. What if advances in our understanding of the neurophysiology of stress lead to substances that can prevent performance loss from raw nerves in the face of raw terror? What if soldiers could be made fearless—or kept alert through sleepless nights—by manipulating their brain chemistry? Doctors who prescribe such pills might try to reassure themselves that the interests of their patients and their country are one and the same. But the possibilities for divergence are endless. Fighters with chemically enhanced courage will take deadly risks that others won't. Advance pharmacological inoculation against fear, anxiety, or exhaustion will surely yield a mix of clinical side-effects and benefits. And what of other possible consequences for patient well-being—say, the lasting feelings of guilt that might follow a fatal miscue induced by chemically induced cocksureness?

All of these possibilities involve clinical relationships, doctor-patient or otherwise, that set national security against clinical subjects' well-being. Some of these possibilities are chilling; drugging people to more easily achieve learned helplessness, for example, would surely constitute torture. Others fall into legal gray areas. There are, for instance, plausible arguments on both sides of the question of whether brain scanning to assess the accuracy of information from captured soldiers would breach the Geneva Conventions. But the disconnect between these possibilities and the Hippocratic ethic of undivided loyalty to patients is a distinct problem—one we'll increasingly face as new technologies emerge. By making it impermissible to admit that clinical relationships can serve society's purposes, the Hippocratic Myth puts this problem beyond the reach of polite discussion.

Where should such a discussion, liberated from the Myth, lead in the national security context? First, as I argued earlier, Hippocratic fidelity isn't at stake absent a personal tie between doctor and clinical subject. When there is a clinical relationship, Hippocratic expectations are in play, and breach of faith is inevitable. Ethicists and lawyers love bright lines between what's permitted and forbidden, but trade-offs between the requisites of national security and trust in medicine are murky and subjective. Still, they're unavoidable—compelling reason to move beyond the Hippocratic Myth. An obvious starting point is prohibition of practices that don't pass muster under human rights law, the laws of war, or other legal safeguards against state excesses. This, of course, begs the question of who decides what the law prohibits, a question made more palpable by the torture memos. It's unrealistic to expect doctors to act as their own lawyers; their dependence on their government for legal advice is part of what made the performance of John Yoo, Jay Bybee, and the other torture memos' authors especially pernicious.[38] But it's reasonable to require that clinical training programs teach human rights basics, so that doctors have some sense of when to say no—or when, at least, to ask hard questions. And it's reasonable for them to insist that their professional associations be prepared to answer these questions and to stand by members who have strong grounds for saying no.

Beyond this starting point, the line between acceptable and improper exploitation of clinical relationships for national security purposes is up for negotiation. Subjective judgment is inevitable—judgment that weighs the urgency of public security concerns against potential harms to trustworthiness in therapeutic relationships. This balancing shouldn't be left to professional societies alone. Sociologists often portray professions as self-governing in ethical matters,[39] but professions formulate their ethics in dialogue with public needs. The Hippocratic pledge of fidelity, as I argued earlier, is an evolving product of this exchange. Its contours change over time in reaction to shifting concerns about professional trustworthiness. Medicine's public roles are part of this dialogue. They're responses to social forces, market pressures, and political decisions, tempered by apprehension over the fragility of patients' trust.[40] Professional associations, sensitive to their members' aims and anxieties, read these social signals and craft ethics policies accordingly. (They can also act quite cynically, as the interrogation saga underscores.) But they don't—and shouldn't—have the final word.

The final word, as a practical matter, is the product of no one actor; it emerges from interplay among public officials, ethics commentators, economic pressures, and cultural influences, as well as professional bodies. Public scandals play a role, by arousing and focusing mass attention, as the ire over Guantanamo and Abu Ghraib illustrates. In the wake of these scandals, clinical assessment of prisoners for the purpose of *lawful* interrogation is widely seen as unethical, although there's not a logical distinction, in my view, between it and assessment of prisoners for forensic purposes. In the end, there often isn't a single ethics outcome. Authorities in position to pronounce on ethical matters commonly take divergent positions. The psychiatry APA's sleight-of-hand "Position Statement" is a case in point—a declamation that scolds Biscuit practitioners while tacitly deferring to the military's more accepting view.

Such divergence often enables us to have it both ways. We skewer doctors for rationing our health care, yet we demand that they do so. At times we condemn them for importing politics into clinical judgment, yet we insist that diagnosis and treatment comport with prevailing moral norms.

But having it both ways spreads confusion, invites distrust, and primes the public for outrage when scandal exposes hypocrisy. What's needed is recognition by all who participate in negotiating the boundaries between social duty and Hippocratic fidelity that hypocrisy of this sort won't do. There's room for different views on where the boundaries should lie, but not for invoking the Hippocratic Myth as a matter of appearances.

I return in the conclusion to the work of negotiating these boundaries as medicine's social roles multiply. But I turn now to another realm in which medicine's public role is expanding: our system of civil and criminal justice. Courts and legislatures are increasingly looking to clinical judgment to make the law's moral choices—choices beyond the scope of diagnostic and therapeutic expertise. And they're asking doctors to use biomedical knowledge for a host of legal purposes far removed from medicine's Hippocratic role.

chapter nine

doing justice?

On a humid July day in 1996, Russell E. Weston appeared at the un-marked entry to CIA headquarters in McLean, Virginia, to tell officials about the "ruby satellite system." He'd created it, he explained. It could stop time, even reverse it. And it could undo events, or replay them an infinite number of times. Worried guards ushered him inside after he told them he was a clone—and a CIA operative nicknamed "The Moon."

In an interview with an agent, he warned of atomic bombs planted around his cabin, told of his close friendship with President Kennedy, and said CIA director James Deutch kept continuous track of his whereabouts with a gold Timex watch. President Clinton, Weston warned, was in on the Kennedy assassination plot and would set off nuclear weapons to stay in power. What happened next is unclear—the CIA keeps mum about its security arrangements. Agency officials gave a heads-up to the Secret Service, routine for threats to the president. But the Secret Service didn't take the threat seriously. Not until October was Weston committed to a state mental hospital, in Montana, after he showed up at a community hospital to com-plain that he'd been brainwashed.

Nearly two months of treatment failed to shake Weston's beliefs. To the contrary, he embellished them, adding details about President Clinton's role in the Kennedy assassination. But fifty-two days after admitting him, his doctors discharged him, deciding that he posed no threat. The thirty-nine-year-old Weston went to Illinois to live with his parents. Once there, he stopped taking his meds, and over the following months, he became concerned about cannibals. They'd taken over the ruby satellite system and were spreading a disease he called "black hava," which caused people's bodies to decay.

Terrified by rotting corpses and the rising power of world cannibalism, he decided to act. He'd regain control of the ruby satellites by getting to the override console on the first floor of the U.S. Capitol, next to the elevators. Weston headed to Washington, convinced that he alone could save America from annihilation. On July 24, 1998, Weston walked through the east entrance to the Capitol, drew a pistol, then rushed toward the offices of Majority Whip Tom DeLay. When two Capitol police officers blocked his way, he fired, fatally wounding both. The dying men returned fire, hitting him in the chest, thigh, and elsewhere.

Weston survived and was charged with capital murder. But he was so obviously crazy that he was immediately sent for psychiatric evaluation, then found incompetent to stand trial—unable, that is, to grasp the meaning of the court proceedings and to assist his lawyers. His prison psychiatrist was a cannibal, he insisted, and so was the judge, who had plans to rig the outcome of his case by putting cannibals on the jury. The men he killed were cannibals as well, bent on keeping him from the satellite system's controls. And they weren't really dead since ruby satellites could reverse time.

In an earlier day, this would have settled the matter, shielding Weston from criminal prosecution but consigning him for a lifetime to a locked psychiatric ward. But the advent of antipsychotic drugs had opened up another possibility: treatment to render a deluded suspect competent to stand trial. Prosecutors demanded this. Weston's lawyers refused, knowing that conviction could mean a death sentence. The matter went to the courts, absent clear legal precedent. Judges had long allowed psychiatrists to forcibly treat patients who posed dangers to life and limb. But Weston's prison psychiatrist, Sally Johnson, said at a hearing that he posed no such risk, at least while locked on the prison's psychiatric unit. And never had a court authorized medicating a defendant against his will solely to make him competent to stand trial.

Weston's lawyers advanced two arguments. First, they said forced medication would deny him a fair trial, since jurors wouldn't see him in an untreated, psychotic state, important to lend support to a plea of insanity. Second, they contended that treatment to make him ready for trial was unethical—a violation of the Hippocratic Oath. Drugging him, they acknowledged, might make him less crazy, anxious, and afraid. But treating him could kill him. The prospect of a death sentence loomed. Paying attention to the drugs' biological efficacy without regard for this life-ending legal consequence would make for perverse parody of the doctor's duty to act for her patient's good.

The judge assigned to Weston's case tried to finesse these arguments by finding him dangerous. But the D.C. Circuit Court of Appeals rejected this gambit, noting Dr. Johnson's testimony to the contrary. The court of appeals told the trial judge, Emmet Sullivan, to decide whether the government could medicate Weston for the sole purpose of making him competent. And the court ordered Judge Sullivan to weigh Weston's medical ethics claim, setting up a confrontation over the propriety of drug treatment for the law's purposes at the price of the patient's well-being. That, at least, was how I saw matters when Weston's lawyers asked me to advise them and to serve as an expert witness on the ethics of treating their client so he could stand trial. Courts might decide either way, but conflict between Hippocratic ideals and the law's purposes was inevitable.

Caught in the middle of this conflict was Sally Johnson, a U.S. Public Health Service psychiatrist assigned to the medical center at Butner, the North Carolina federal prison to which Weston had been sent. Johnson hadn't originally planned on making psychotic killers her life's work. As a child, she'd wanted to be a pianist. By her mid-teens, this ambition lay in the past. "I went to medical school because I really didn't know what I wanted to do," she told me years after we tangled in Judge Sullivan's courtroom over medical ethics and Weston's fate. But she went in all the way, passing up four years of college in favor of an accelerated program at Jefferson Medical College that awarded her a medical degree five years after finishing high school. Johnson covered her own costs with scholarships, including one from the

Public Health Service that required her to join it after her residency. And she fell in love with psychiatry. Or, rather, she says, psychiatry fell for her. "It seems that psychiatry likes me, in a weird way. People approach me and tell me about their lives. . . . I really like really crazy people, and they seem to be really comfortable with me."

On the computer software that changes medical students' life courses by matching them to internships and residencies, Johnson ranked Duke highly. Duke did the same for her. "I wanted to go south," she said. "And, lo and behold, . . . they were opening a new federal prison, and Duke was involved in trying to help them get the mental health unit going. . . . There were really crazy people there." So she went to Duke for her residency, then stayed in North Carolina for her career. Since the Public Health Service provides doctors to federal prisons, she could do her payback at Butner, the new facility Duke had helped to set up. Johnson loved the work. She became nationally renowned as a forensic evaluator—the government's go-to person for a succession of celebrity criminals with psychiatric issues. They included Theodore Kaczynski, the "Unabomber"; John Hinckley, President Reagan's would-be assassin; and Jim Bakker, the televangelist; as well as Weston. They fascinated her, as did the questions the law put to her about personal accountability.

And the awkward question of conflict between Hippocratic commitment and the law's purposes didn't seem, to her, a problem at all. She averted the question by treating the law's requirements as givens—matters over which she had no responsibility, even when they turned on what she said. "I try never to enter into being the legal decision maker," she told me. "That isn't my role." That's how she saw Weston's fitness to stand trial. He had a right and a duty to participate in the legal process. Her responsibility was to get him ready. "I'm a clinician who is trying to understand illness as it fits into getting on that playing field. If you're stuck in a system where you need to be playing on that field, then I'd like to see you be as sound as you can on that field. That's because the requirement is to play."

Federal law framed the question of a prison doctor's role in ambiguous terms. The Supreme Court had held that treatment must be "medically appropriate" or in an inmate's "best medical interest," even when given to make him less dangerous to others.[1] Later decisions had hinted at the possibility of forced medication to restore competence but maintained the "best medical interest" requirement. What, though, did "best medical interest" mean? Did it refer only to a treatment's biological impact—its side-effects and relief of target symptoms? Or did it compel attention to life circumstances, including potential legal fallout?

For doctors taught, as most are, to consider the whole patient, not just one or another organ system, answering this question is easy. Life consequences count as much as biological systems, an ideal often honored in the breach by medical specialists but still a core precept of clinical care. That's the argument Weston's lawyers pressed to support their claim that forcible medication to make their client competent in a capital case couldn't possibly be in his "best medical interest." A court might command treatment for the law's purposes, but the doctor asked to carry out the order would face a conflict between her responsibilities to the state and to her patient, even if the prescribed treatment were, in a biological sense, right.

Sally Johnson insisted otherwise. On the witness stand at a July 2000 hearing, she was asked whether she saw any conflict between her duties to Weston and to the law. "No, I don't," she told the court, several times. True, she said, there were "multiple rationales for medication," including "treatment of his symptom picture" and "restoration of his competency." And competency, she acknowledged, was "the principle reason for medication"—"that's what he was sent here for treatment to accomplish."[2]

Weston's lawyers grasped this opportunity—a crack in the facade—an admission that Dr. Johnson's role wasn't purely patient focused. "As his treating physician," public defender A. J. Kramer asked, "your duty is solely to the patient?" "Not in this case," Johnson replied. "Because he is there only by order of the Court. He's not a voluntary patient." Kramer made his move: "The Hippocratic Oath, the central tenet, is first do no harm to the patient?"[3] Dr. Johnson: "That's one of the tenets, yes." Kramer pressed: "Do you see a conflict in your loyalties to Mr. Weston as opposed to your duties with the Court?" "No," Dr. Johnson persevered. "I see him as suffering from a mental illness that requires treatment for alleviation of his symptom picture, and I feel no conflict in providing that treatment to him if I'm authorized."

At this point, Kramer noted that Weston had *refused* medication upon being found competent to make medical decisions shortly after his arrest. Wasn't Johnson, as his doctor, bound to follow this? No, she said, because "the Court committed him to me for treatment"—treatment "necessary" for "restoration of competence." "I guess that's my point," Kramer answered, underscoring the divergence between her caregiving and law enforcement roles. "You think treatment is necessary to restore him to competency, even though that might lead to his execution." Dr. Johnson pushed back, insisting on a marriage between the law's purposes and her patient's interests: "I'm tasked by the Court . . . , whether it is a potential death penalty case or not, to provide treatment for the mental illness in an effort to restore the defendant's competency to stand trial, and that's to offer them their full involvement in the legal process, to maximize the outcome in their favor."

This last claim was implausible. There are surely defendants for whom going to trial won't "maximize the outcome in their favor." Weston almost certainly was one. The Capitol shootings had drawn the outrage of law enforcement officers and others nationwide, he'd clearly fired the fatal shots, and an insanity plea was hardly a sure thing. He stood no small chance of being executed. And the question of whether one or another legal strategy might "maximize the outcome" in his favor was one for his lawyers, not his (or the state's) doctor. They're "tasked by the Court" and our system of justice with the balancing of legal probabilities on their client's behalf. In her effort to deny her own role conflict, Johnson intruded on their responsibilities.

Johnson *could,* at this point, have conceded that the demands the criminal law put upon her were in conflict with her caregiving role. But the Hippocratic Myth stood in the way. It drove her to depict her court-centered work in patient-centered terms, so as to keep from admitting to herself or others that her clinical efforts often compromised her patients' good. Such an admission might have been the first step toward striking a balance between patient-centered purposes and the law's expectations. The Hippocratic Myth, though, is an absolute—it doesn't admit of such balancing. Doctors who openly offend against the Myth imperil their professional standing and their sense of self. Like others in this book, Dr. Johnson arrived at an understanding of her role that elided the conflict she faced daily, between society's demands and the Hippocratic ideal. An irony embedded in her understanding is that it asserted a political and moral premise: that people charged with crimes have a responsibility to submit to the law's processes. Most people agree with this proposition; Johnson was far from being a rogue moral actor. But by incorporating this premise into her understanding of Weston's "best medical interest," she became a moral *enforcer*, a function at odds with the Hippocratic ideal.

Craziness and Responsibility

Doctors act as moral arbiters and enforcers across an expanding array of legal settings, often going far beyond the boundaries of what science shows. They've long opined on legal competence—to sign contracts, write wills, and make health care decisions, as well as to stand trial. Their clinical expertise plays a role: Interviewing, physical exams, and lab tests guide appraisals of cognitive capability, and knowledge of diagnostic criteria enables them to fit their findings into disease categories. But the leap of inference from diagnosis to diminished competence is a leap powered by moral judgment. It's a no-brainer that Weston's schizophrenic symptoms, including his conviction that Judge Sullivan and Dr. Johnson were cannibals, left him unable to adequately understand the trial process or the charges against him. The reasons why it's a no-brainer, though, are moral, not scientific. Bizarre beliefs of the sort he held, beliefs characteristic of schizophrenia, fall below our consensus about the level of understanding necessary to participate in the legal process.

But higher levels of functioning can fall into morally contested zones. Consider, for example, a grandmother with Alzheimer's disease who suffers from profound defects in memory and cognition, as well as the emotional lability—the spells of sadness, fear, and rage—that contribute to making Alzheimer's a nightmare for friends and loved ones. Suppose, out of ire over imagined neglect, she redraws her will to cut out her daughter, instead bestowing her largess on a man she's just met who visits her often, tells her she's lovely, and makes her feel good about herself. She dies, the will is found, and the shocked daughter sues, claiming Mom wasn't competent to revise it. There's enough money at stake to pay for a parade of neurologists and psychiatrists to opine in court on the question, citing sundry Alzheimer's symptoms. But at what point should slips of understanding and surges of feeling negate Mom's legal right to dispose of her assets as she pleases? At what point must she, or anyone, surrender her autonomy—her freedom to participate in social and economic life as an adult, and her responsibility for her actions?

That's a moral matter, made more nuanced by the truth that all of us act on our passions[4] and make myriad cognitive errors.[5] The law allows us to act stupidly, vengefully, and lovingly—and holds us accountable when we don't hew to its standards. When doctors distinguish between competent and incompetent states of mind, they're issuing moral judgments as to when cognitive lapses and rushes of feeling should lead to limits on freedom and responsibility.

The same is the case when psychiatrists speak to the question of criminal responsibility, as they have since the early nineteenth century when defendants have claimed insanity. Madness as a defense to criminal charges has origins in ancient law. Greeks, Romans, Hebrews, and Muslims variously treated states of unreason and imbecility as grounds for relieving people of responsibility for wrongdoing or withholding punishment. The early common law of England emphasized the question of understanding. By the 1500s, English judges were asking whether purportedly insane defendants understood "good and evil." In 1724, one "Justice Tracy" set out this test in memorable fashion, calling for an inquiry into whether "a man [is] totally deprived of his understanding and memory, so as not to know what he is doing, no more than an infant, a brute, or a wild beast."[6]

In what came to be known as the "wild beast" test, doctors only occasionally played a role. Jurors and judges assessed the accused's "understanding and memory"; medical diagnosis wasn't necessary. Not until the early 1800s did mental illness become a prerequisite for excuse by reason of insanity. In the celebrated affair that made this official, a paranoid named Daniel M'Naghten became convinced that the British prime minister, Robert Peel, meant him harm. M'Naghten shot Peel dead, or so he mistakenly thought; Peel's unlucky private secretary was the victim instead. M'Naghten pled insanity and prevailed, angering Queen Victoria and many others. The House of Lords demanded that the judges come in person to explain themselves—by American standards, a shocking breach of separation-of-powers. The judges did so, in a way that restricted the reach of the insanity defense by requiring mental illness. To establish the defense, they said, "it must be conclusively proved that, at the time of the committing of the act, the party accused was laboring under such a defect of reason, *from the disease of the mind,* as not to know the nature and quality of the act he was doing; or if he did know it, that he did not know what he was doing was wrong."[7]

Psychiatrists, or "alienists" (as psychiatrists were called in the nineteenth century), became courtroom regulars, speaking to the question of whether "disease of the mind" was present, as well as whether the "disease" caused a sufficient "defect of reason." The diagnostic categories of the day thus became moral categories—realms of unaccountability mapped by doctors sure that they were practicing clinical science. Abnormal "manifestations of the intellect and . . . sentiments," wrote Isaac Ray, the century's preeminent authority on forensic psychiatry, are "dependent upon . . . abnormal conditions of the brain." Brain dissections by "eminent observers," he decreed, "have placed it beyond a doubt . . . that deviations from the healthy structure are generally presented in the brains of insane subjects."[8]

To be sure, once we shunt aside supernatural explanations, all "manifestations" of the mind reflect the functioning of the brain. But that's hardly the same as saying that the diagnostic *categories* doctors adopt are objectively derivable from brain biology. Diagnostic categories group signs and symptoms for sundry reasons, including availability of effective treatments, understandings of disease mechanisms, and beliefs about what is and isn't normal. *All* behavior is biologically caused in some fashion; treating diagnostic groupings as grounds for excuse is thus biologically arbitrary. Picking and choosing among biological causes—counting some as excuses while disregarding others—is a moral endeavor, not a scientific one. Empowering doctors to do the picking and choosing—by deferring to their diagnostic categories—makes them into practitioners of public morals, under the guise of clinical expertise.

That they've sometimes practiced public morals with imperiousness is underscored by Ray's declaration that dissections have shown "beyond a doubt" that "deviations from healthy structure" are found in the brains of the criminally insane. What was "beyond a doubt" to Ray would later be thoroughly disproven. None of the "deviations" found by nineteenth-century neuropathologists correlated with abnormal behavior of any sort—neither with criminal conduct nor with psychiatric symptoms that fit the diagnostic categories of the day. The century saw a succession of efforts to establish such connections, most famously by practitioners of phrenology, who cataloged variations in skull shape and purported to tie them to character. Proponents of phrenology contended in courtrooms, pressing theories of racial difference as well as mental deficiency, until their ideas wore out their welcome as the century came to an end.

Later developments further expanded the role of doctors as arbiters of criminal accountability. Ray and others pressed the claim that the mere presence of mental disease should excuse any criminal act caused by the disease. Whether the accused knew "the nature and quality of the act" or understood that "what he was doing was wrong" was beside the point. Judges began to buy in. As one early-adopter put it, "when disease is the propelling, uncontrollable power, the man is as innocent as the weapon."[9]

Over the course of the late nineteenth and early twentieth centuries, courts endorsed this proposition in varying forms, dispensing with inquiries into knowledge of right and wrong. The aptly-named "Group for the Advancement of Psychiatry" celebrated in 1954, when the Court of Appeals for the D.C. Circuit held simply that "an accused is not criminally responsible if his unlawful act was the product of mental disease or mental defect."[10] (This is the approach the Group had urged.) A few years later, the influential American Law Institute urged an only slightly restrained version. It was quickly adopted by federal judges and many state courts. An accused shouldn't be held "responsible for criminal conduct," the Institute said, "if at the time of such conduct *as the result of mental disease or defect* he lacks substantial capacity either to appreciate the criminality of his conduct *or* to conform his conduct to the requirements of law."[11]

The Institute's approach preserved *M'Naghten*'s reference to appreciation of right and wrong in vestigial form only. It invited doctors to opine on whether mental illness deprived defendants of "substantial capacity" to "conform" their actions to the law, and it allowed judges and jurors to excuse criminal acts on this basis. Medicine had achieved sovereignty over the question of criminal responsibility. Doctors exercised this power collectively, by hewing to agreed-upon disease categories, and individually, through case-by-case judgments as to whether defendants could have complied with the law.

In so doing, doctors rendered moral verdicts invisibly, even disingenuously. At no point did psychiatry make a moral case for counting biological causes of behavior as excuses only if they fit the field's diagnostic categories. If all behavior arises from brain physiology, why should one biological cause be privileged over another as an excuse on the basis of a diagnostic label? What about social influences on people's actions? These play out through brain biology, so why shouldn't they excuse criminal acts? David Bazelon, author of the 1954 D.C. Circuit opinion excusing acts that were the "product" of mental illness, later urged exactly this, calling for recognition of "rotten social background" as an excuse.[12] Philosophers, legal scholars, and the lay public have long struggled over how to square scientific understandings of behavior with the fixing of blame. If all human acts have knowable causes, isn't blame always unfair? To answer yes would be to render criminal responsibility unjust per se, a radical proposition for the governance of human affairs.

We're hardly ready to embrace this disruptive notion. So we muddle through the contradictions between brain science and blame, open to what philosophers, religious leaders, and physicians have to say, but insistent on popular sovereignty over the limits of culpability. In democratic societies, these limits are for voters and jurors, judges, and elected officials to set. They're not for psychiatrists (or other physicians) to draw covertly, under cover of claims about the objectivity of diagnosis.

Likewise, the conceit that clinical science can distinguish between defendants who could and couldn't have "conform[ed] . . . to the requirements of law" covers over the moral judgment this distinction demands. To say that a person could have done something he or she didn't do makes no scientific sense. As artificial intelligence researcher Douglas Hofstadter has pointed out, "[I]t is obvious that anything that didn't happen didn't happen. There aren't degrees of 'didn't-happen-ness.'"[13]

One might, to be sure, imagine counterfactuals. Had 537 fewer Floridians voted for Ralph Nader instead of Al Gore in November 2000, George Bush wouldn't have become president. Had baseball umpire Jim Joyce not botched a call at first base with two outs in the ninth inning on June 2, 2010, Detroit Tigers pitcher Armando Galarraga would have been credited with a perfect game (video replays showed the runner was out by several feet; Joyce called him safe). And had Joyce not apologized tearfully on television, exclaiming, "I just cost that kid a perfect game" (and had Galarraga not accepted the apology and given him a hug), the two wouldn't have been linked thereafter as icons of grace.[14]

These things almost didn't happen, or so it seems. But consider another "almost," recounted by Hofstadter: "A friend said to me, 'My uncle was almost President of the U.S.' 'Really?' I said. 'Sure,' he replied, 'he was skipper of the *PT 108*.' (John F. Kennedy was skipper of the *PT 109*.)" This is funny because it's preposterous. But as Hofstadter notes, the preposterousness lies in the mind, not the facts. Neither Al Gore nor the skipper of the *PT 108* became president. We can more easily imagine Gore being sworn in, but it's equally impossible to undo either outcome. It's likewise impossible (absent the ruby satellite system's ability to reverse time) to undo a murder, whether committed in response to a paranoid delusion or in cold blood. Brain biology, influenced by environmental and genetic factors, can in theory explain both. The webs of causation are complex but inexorable.

To conclude that a defendant could or couldn't have "conform[ed] his conduct to the requirements of law"—after he has failed to do so—is to render a judgment that makes no sense in scientific terms. It's a *moral* assessment—a judgment about what society should expect a person to refrain from doing, given the circumstances.[15] Such judgments may themselves be biologically driven: There's growing evidence that we (and other primates) are hardwired to form beliefs about personal culpability.[16] But they're not judgments that doctors have special expertise to make. They're judgments that arise from popular sensibilities—judgments that, in a democracy, aren't for medicine to issue under the false cover of science.

After a District of Columbia jury found John Hinckley not guilty by reason of insanity in 1982, popular sensibilities asserted themselves. Within a few months of the reading of the verdict, the U.S. House and Senate held hearings on the insanity defense—hearings that cast the courts as having allowed psychiatry to run amok over personal responsibility. Over the next several years, Congress and most states trimmed back the defense, dispensing with formulations that excused crimes based on psychiatric explanations of cause. Congress retreated to a variant of *M'Naghten,* limiting the defense to those who, "as a result of a severe mental disease or defect, [were] unable to appreciate the nature and quality or the wrongfulness of [their] acts."[17] Psychiatric diagnosis remained a prerequisite, keeping mental health professionals in the picture as arbiters of culpability. But the question of defendants' appreciation of their actions—and of right and wrong—had become equally central. Medical accounts of a criminal act's causes would no longer do.

Had Russell Weston gone to trial, it's hardly clear that he'd have surmounted this legal hurdle. Dr. Johnson or one of her colleagues might well have argued that he understood he was shooting to kill and knew doing so was wrong. A defense psychiatrist might have answered that Weston thought ruby satellites could reverse time, bringing the dead officers back to life, and that he believed the threat of cannibalism called for drastic action. How jurors might have resolved the matter is an open question.

It's a question that, in all likelihood, will never be answered. After the July 2000 hearing on whether Weston should be medicated against his will to make him competent to stand trial, Judge Sullivan ruled for the prosecution and ordered him treated. A D.C. Circuit Court of Appeals panel upheld Sullivan, dismissing the Hippocratic ethics concerns his lawyers raised as not "relevant." Antipsychotic drugs were "medically appropriate" for his "condition," the panel said, and the prospect of his execution was beside the point. The U.S. Supreme Court declined to hear Weston's appeal, and Dr. Johnson began treatment, confident of the "high likelihood"[18] of success. The D.C. Circuit panel had expressed equal confidence in its medication order, concluding that there was only a "small possibility that antipsychotic medication will not make Weston competent for trial."[19] For the next several years, prison doctors tried a succession of drug combinations. None worked. Weston remained consumed by fear of cannibals and the ruby satellite system's powers. His lawyers and doctors became part of his delusions. As this book went to press, he remained in Butner's prison hospital, unfit for trial and unlikely ever to be freed.

The role of doctors as arbiters on the law's behalf extends far beyond the realms of mental competence and criminal responsibility. Physicians opine on most of the more than 2 million social security disability claims filed in the United States each year, almost half of which were granted in 2009.[20] The Social Security Act requires, for an award of benefits, a "medically determinable physical or mental impairment" that's expected to kill the claimant or last for at least a year. This impairment, moreover, must result in an "inability to engage in any substantial gainful activity."[21] To this end, doctors list symptoms and diagnoses, judge levels of disability, and convey their conclusions to claims examiners and administrative law judges in writing and at hearings. Detailed regulations prescribe criteria for awarding benefits, cabining the discretion of doctors and claims examiners. But there's an irreducible realm of subjective judgment about the severity of people's symptoms and their ability to work. Embedded in these judgments are premises about the hardships the state should expect citizens to endure and the extent to which people should fend for themselves.

For disability applicants and their loved ones, the stakes are often enormous. Denials can mean impoverishment and even homelessness for claimants and their families. And the impact of a denial often ripples outward— to parents and to adult children—and to aunts, uncles, and cousins—who strain their finances to try to help. That the doctors who render decisive opinions are most often the claimants' treating physicians can tear clinical trust asunder. Doctors can develop a toxic suspiciousness, and patients can become resentful in return. I recall filling out innumerable social security disability forms as an exhausted resident, for patients who lacked health insurance and were therefore stuck with me. I saw their desperation, I was at times the object of their anger, and, more often than I'd care to admit, I harbored doubts about what they told me.

The Lawless World of Child Custody

Millions of Americans are affected in life-changing fashion by the opinions mental health professionals render in child custody cases. Each year, more than a million children suffer the breakup of their families through divorce. An uncounted number of additional children, surely in the hundreds of thousands, endure the separation of unmarried parents. It's been estimated that nearly half of all babies born to married parents will lose their families to divorce before they turn eighteen. For children born out of wedlock, the prospect of parental breakup is much higher. Children lose parents or find their relationships with one or both parents utterly transformed. Fathers and mothers are suddenly threatened with the loss of their children, and their roles in their children's lives often shrink dramatically.

During the early years of the American republic, resolution of such cases was predictable. Divorce was rare. When it happened, fathers almost always received sole custody. They had property rights to their children; mothers didn't.[22] Over the course of the nineteenth century, this approach was slowly supplanted by a preference for mothers. The so-called "tender years" doctrine held that women were, by nature or God's gift, more affectionate and otherwise better-suited to care for children, especially those younger than age thirteen. "Tender years" prevailed through the mid-twentieth century, buttressed by medical theories that cast women as too weak for the rigors of the workplace but more nurturing than their menfolk at home.

Although the sex bias embedded in these legal doctrines was blatant, this bias was, at least, honest. First men, then women, were favored as parents. And these dubious doctrines yielded easily foreseen results. Judges could apply them—and did—without exercising broad discretion or sweating the case-by-case details. Health professionals were rarely involved. Their role was limited to the diagnosis and documentation of serious illness—illness disabling enough to upset the presumptions of paternal or maternal custody that these doctrines imposed. Such custody battles as did occur were fought on moralistic grounds. Men challenged the "fitness" of their former wives, alleging sexual license or other forms of turpitude. Women questioned men's willingness to provide for their children and to teach them about right and wrong.

The 1960s and 1970s wrought radical change. Divorce rates soared. Women rejected the limits on their life chances outside the home that the "tender years" doctrine (and its supporting biological theories) implied. Men insisted on a larger role in the rearing of their children, both within their marriages and after divorce. Courts backed away from overt sex bias in the law of family dissolution, preferring doctrinal formulations that promised gender equity. The content-free "best interest of the child" standard replaced "tender years," freeing family law from the stigma of overt bias but forcing judges to award custody without the guidance of law.[23] By the mid-1980s, nearly every state had abandoned "tender years." Custody contests became a free-fire realm—a realm without rules, beset by raw passions.

Into this lawless void, mental health professionals entered eagerly. The pioneers were two renowned Freudians, psychiatrist Albert Solnit and Sigmund Freud's daughter and disciple, Anna. Working with a legal scholar, Joseph Goldstein, who himself trained as a psychoanalyst (and treated patients in his faculty office at Yale Law School), the two formulated the theory that every young child has a "psychological parent"—a primary caregiver on whom the child counts for affection, security, and satisfaction of life's basic needs.[24] Tearing a child away from her "psychological parent," Goldstein once told a court (in a custody case), would have lifelong, shattering impact, leaving her "damaged and bruised," with "a sense of rejection and distrust about the external world."[25] It would interrupt the process of "internaliz[ing] the parent," critical to a child's ability to venture confidently into the outside world.[26] In custody contests, therefore, the court's task was clear-cut: to identify the "psychological parent," award him or her full custody, and get other, intruding would-be caregivers out of the way. To this end, psychiatrists and psychologists offered themselves as experts to divorce lawyers and family courts. This offer was eagerly embraced.

There was no more science behind the "psychological parent" proposition (and Goldstein's gloomy prediction) than there was behind phrenologists' theories of skull shape. There were no large-scale field studies of parent-child relationships; nor was there anything resembling rigorous measurement of parenting outcomes.[27] What "proved" the proposition to its proponents was an act of imagination, captured by Goldstein in his elegy to Anna Freud upon her passing: "Miss Freud taught us to put childish things before, not behind, us. She taught us to place ourselves in a child's skin, to try to think a child's thoughts and feel a child's feelings about being 'removed from a known environment to an unknown one,' about his 'residence being divided evenly between two warring parents' or about having to visit an absent parent on 'prescribed days and hours.'"[28]

It's pedestrian to point out that Anna Freud had no way of knowing whether she was feeling a child's feelings—and that this act of imagination disregarded the down-the-line benefits of involving both parents in a child's daily life. It's pedestrian—but essential to an understanding of the power mental health professionals began to assert as arbiters of family structure.

That Goldstein, Freud, and Solnit knew they were asserting power (and didn't shy from it) is plain. In a 1966 letter to Solnit and Yale Law's dean about a possible faculty appointment, Freud expressed excitement about "[t]he plan of drafting a model code of procedure for the disposition of children."[29] Four years earlier, at her first meeting with Goldstein, she'd let him in on what so excited her about their possible collaboration: "Because my father as a young man wished, for a time, to study law. He had always hoped to establish a rapprochement between psychoanalysis and law."[30] And in his 1982 elegy upon her passing, Goldstein spoke with gratitude about her impact on family law: "As lawyers, legislators, law teachers, and judges, we continue to draw on what she taught."[31]

What she taught enabled custody courts to stay, on the surface, sex neutral while putting into effect a strong preference for mothers. True, fathers were and are the main caregivers in some families, but women do most of the hands-on parenting of infants and young children. Later research would show a tendency for men's time with their children to rise steadily, starting in the preschool years, toward equivalence with women's parenting time as children entered their teens.[32] Other research—not done by psychoanalysts—would show that highly-engaged fathers enhance their children's academic performance, self-confidence, and social adjustment.[33] The Goldstein, Freud, and Solnit psychological parent formulation cut off these possibilities with a preemptive strike. It was winner-take-all, and the winner was usually Mom, based on her larger early-childhood role. "Tender years," in other words, enjoyed life after death. It was smuggled into custody cases by mental health professionals long after the courts had formally abandoned it.

For mothers in the midst of custody warfare, this was a happy circumstance—a strategic advantage camouflaged by the law's purported neutrality and psychiatry's (and psychology's) patina of professional expertise. But for women intent on breaking from sex stereotypes and pursuing their career dreams, the "psychological parent" thesis was a rebuke. It suggested that they should stay home with their children so as not to leave them "damaged and bruised," with feelings of abandonment and distrust toward the world. Conversely, it freed most men from fatherly obligations, on the ground that they were of marginal import to their children and, after divorce, should get out of the way.

Custody evaluators who invoked the psychological parent proposition practiced cultural politics—conservative politics that pushed back against women's efforts to combine motherhood with career and men's yearning to make fatherhood more central to their lives. More than that, these mental health professionals made social policy. Especially in the inner city and other places where out-of-wedlock births were pandemic, they raised barriers to fathers' remaining in the picture. Once the question of custody and child support reached court, a father's initial absence became a legal barrier to his reengagement. His task was to pay; his parenting role was peripheral.

Research would later show the obvious: Absent fathers are more likely to become "deadbeat dads" than are fathers who participate in their children's lives.[34] Thus, pushing fathers to the periphery not only shortchanged kids developmentally; it left them and their mothers materially worse off. This, the forensic evaluators who followed Goldstein, Freud, and Solnit utterly ignored.

By the mid-1980s, participation of psychiatrists and psychologists in custody disputes had become routine. Adherents to the psychological parent proposition were the pioneers, but believers in other models of parenting and its dysfunctions enthusiastically offered their services. Divorce lawyers shopped for favorable experts, clients fearful of losing their children paid willingly, and courts looking for impartial guidance appointed their own mental health professionals. In other fields of law, judges aggressively policed the admission of experts' conclusions, reading rules of evidence to require that they have some scientific basis.[35] But custody contests were a science-free zone. Courts clueless about how to answer the lawless best-interest-of-the-child question listened to custody evaluators' conclusions about who would make the best parent, then typically rubber-stamped their recommended results.

That there isn't a "science" of custody evaluation has been long recognized by researchers but ignored by the courts.[36] About all that can be said for sure about outcomes for children is that exposure to parental conflict predicts poorer emotional health and school performance.[37] A mother's or father's serious mental illness also puts a child at psychological (and even physical) risk, absent the stabilizing influence of a coparent. So psychiatrists can contribute to custody decisions in evidence-based fashion by assessing parents for mental illness. Their experience as observers of people might even empower them to spot behavior that sparks conflict. But how to balance the risks of a parent's mental illness against the positives he or she offers—and how to go from observations of button-pushing behavior to recommendations about who should raise a child—are questions of value, beyond the reach of clinical expertise.

Answers to these and other questions of value animate clinicians' custody recommendations. Examples include the choice between a mother's tenderness and a father's resolve, between one parent's emphasis on academics and the other's focus on sports or social life, and between parents' lifestyles and faith commitments. The cultural issues that divide Americans when they vote, pray, and connect with others in person or online are ammunition in custody warfare—and grist for custody evaluators' judgments.

These judgments are typically decisive. Aware that judges expect clinical evaluations in contested cases,[38] lawyers for both parents usually agree upon a mental health professional (unless the court selects one). And knowing that judges generally go with the evaluator's recommendations, lawyers typically tell "losing" clients to accept this result rather than chancing trial. After the evaluation comes in, the parties customarily settle. For all but the wealthiest of warring parents, economics compels this. Going to trial is commonly a six-figure proposition—tens of thousands of dollars for legal fees and a second evaluator (often less credible to the court than the one agreed to by both parties). Weighed against the improbability of winning, this impoverishing expenditure can seem an act of madness.[39]

Custody evaluators are thus virtually immunized from close scrutiny of their cultural and moral premises. Since custody trials are unusual, cross-examination of evaluators in court is rare. When parties settle before trial, evaluators' cultural and moral preferences shape parenting plans sight unseen. In many jurisdictions, moreover, doctors who perform these evaluations are immune from malpractice suits. And evaluations typically are kept secret after custody is resolved. Judges "seal" court records. Parties that settle commit to keeping these reports confidential. They fear humiliating revelations and future cycles of family recrimination. It's thus nearly impossible to hold evaluators accountable, whether through suits for malpractice, professional disciplinary action, or compilation of *Consumer Reports*–style reviews of past performance.

This freedom from scrutiny also empowers custody evaluators to usurp the courts' role as finders of fact. Casting their work as clinical assessment, evaluators interview parents and children, therapists and lovers, employers and teachers, and just about anyone else they choose. The law's usual safeguards against personal intrusion don't apply: There is no medical confidentiality, for example, when the custody evaluator calls. Nor do the rules of evidence or due process apply. Evaluators make judgments about who did what to whom and whose fault it was under cover of supposed clinical expertise. There aren't rules against hearsay, nor rights to cross-examine disparaging claims, nor chances to put half-truths into context. Instead, courts treat evaluators' *judgments* as "evidence"—evidence worthy of extra weight because of their expertise.[40]

Fred and Ally Go to War

The secrecy that surrounds custody evaluations has stymied public discussion of the power these evaluators hold. The several critiques of custody evaluation published in the research literature contain no case examples—no reports by evaluators who rendered judgment beyond the scope of their expertise. But reports I've obtained, on condition of anonymity, show how far some evaluators are willing to go.[41] The custody contest that began when Fred Russo told his wife, Ally,[42] over breakfast that he wanted a divorce offers an illustration.

As with such a moment in any marriage, much had preceded it—a *Rashomon* of rival narratives not possible for an outsider to parse. The couple had met almost exactly 20 years before, in 1983, on a touch-football field in D.C. Fred was playing; Ally took an interest. Eyes met, and passions surged. Twenty-something sensuality matured into romance. They found deeper commonalities: parents' emotional troubles, family strife, and dreams of a more secure adult life. And they discovered differences: her effusiveness and adventurous spirit (she'd lived in a dozen countries as a child and loved connecting with people from diverse cultures) and his self-contained manner and plan to take up the suburban lifestyle of his family of origin.

Fred finished law school in Washington; Ally traveled the world as a flight attendant for Pan Am. After he graduated, he took a job with a supermarket chain in New Jersey, where he'd grown up and his extended family still lived. By 1987, they were married, with an infant son, and living in a north Jersey suburb. A daughter, then another son soon followed. So did rising tension. Ally, who'd become a stay-at-home mom, felt stifled by suburban living. Fred was unhappy with his work; Ally, unhappy with his long hours. And as their oldest son, Raymond, moved beyond his toddler years, troubles emerged. There were angry outbursts and failures to follow social cues. At school, he didn't focus as some thought he should. Fred thought he needed firmer discipline; Ally took a more tender approach. Over time, positions hardened, as did Fred's and Ally's feelings toward each other.

Mental health professionals entered the picture, as marriage counselors and personal therapists. Diagnoses proliferated—"attention deficit hyperactivity disorder" (ADHD) and "Asperger's syndrome" (a mild form of autism) for Raymond, "adult attention deficit disorder" for Fred, and anxiety and depression for Ally. And there was violence, which grew worse as Raymond moved through his teen years. Knives were drawn on a few occasions. A phone was ripped from a wall. Punches were thrown, as were household objects. Ally's mouth was once bloodied, as was Raymond's. At least twice, Fred summoned the police; once, they placed Raymond under arrest. Through the he-said-she-said haze, it's difficult to point to perpetrators and victims, though it appears from court documents Ally shared with me that Fred initiated more than his proportionate share. Fred also aroused Raymond's ire repeatedly by videotaping him, something Fred claimed had a therapeutic purpose—to show Raymond how bad his behavior had become. Within the family, alliances formed and faced off. Raymond's sister, Ana, three years younger, leaned toward her dad. Raymond saw himself as his mom's protector, and his brother Jack, seven years his junior and very much his admirer, sided with the two of them.

When, on March 1, 2003, at 7 AM, Fred told Ally he wanted a divorce, Ally was devastated. Raymond was outraged. "He left us, he abandoned us," Ana later recalled Raymond's saying. Fred moved out on the twentieth anniversary of the day they'd met, and Ally made plans to move with the children to Washington. She had friends, family, and job prospects there, and she craved the city's more cosmopolitan environment. She'd learned of several outstanding special education programs, better for Raymond, she figured, than anything she'd found in New Jersey. And she wanted out of New Jersey, away from Fred and his family and her memories of their marital journey from romance to despair.

But this would have left Fred a visitor in the lives of his children—an occasional weekend dad. He chose to fight. So did Ally. And so began the worst kind of custody war—a struggle over a move-away, in which possibilities for compromise are all but eliminated by the fact that children can't go back and forth between schools, daily or weekly, to accommodate the breakup of their families. Ally sought the court's permission to take the children to Washington; Fred asked the court to say no on the ground that the kids needed their father. The lawyers agreed on a custody evaluator, clinical psychologist Jonathan Elson, who interviewed the parties and their three children for more than twenty hours, then questioned their therapists, Ally's potential employer, and others.

Had the case played out as custody matters typically do, Elson would have made his "recommendations," then the parties would have settled the case by adopting them. Ally would have lost her move-away bid, or Fred would have lost his children, based on Elson's life-changing call. And his report, like others I sought out for this chapter, would have been confidential by court order or the terms of the settlement. But when Elson opined that Ally shouldn't be allowed to move with the children, she refused to go along. She hired new lawyers and additional evaluators. Fred fought back. There were endless court dates, depositions, and appointments with therapists recommended by each other. The couple's bills for lawyers, evaluators, and assorted therapists soared, to more than $2 million, Ally estimates, over the next several years.

This legal frenzy permits a glimpse at the content of custody evaluations. No settlement or court order requires that Elson's be kept secret. His written assessment is more thorough than most I've reviewed—sixty-three single-spaced pages reporting on his interviews and rendering "clinical" judgments. There are occasional references to diagnoses made by the health care providers he questioned, but there's no claim that illness of any kind makes Ally or Fred unfit as parents. There are, aplenty, findings of fact that don't draw on clinical expertise. Elson concluded, for example, that

Ally "had all three children phone [Fred] to negotiate his parenting time with them, as if they were Ally's advocates." According to Elson: "On occasions that [Fred] has come to pick up the younger children, [Ally] has sent [Raymond] to the car with the message that '[Jack] hates you and doesn't want to go with you.'" And once, Elson wrote, when Raymond agreed by phone to spend several weekdays instead of a weekend with Fred, Ally "started shouting (with Fred still on the line), 'Why did you do that? This will ruin our case.'" What were Elson's grounds for deciding that Ally had done these things? He doesn't say. The reader, it seems, is supposed to take these findings as givens.

In the mad world of custody warfare, such findings are explosive. Custody combat's prime directives are to keep children out of the crossfire and to create "facts on the ground," since courts don't like to disrupt existing arrangements. So, in no-holds-barred custody battles, parties try to portray their opponents as putting the kids in the middle. They also look to keep the current schedule in line with their legal goals. But if they're caught acting tactically, they pay in credibility, and they invite the perception that they're willing to use their children as weapons. So being seen as stoking a child's bad feelings toward the other parent—or as blocking a schedule swap to keep Dad from winning weekday time[43]—just plain looks awful.

Elson also parsed language, playing both judge and interrogator of everyday contradictions. He pressed Ally to "reconcile [her] seemingly inconsistent statements": She had, for example, described her brother as "completely supportive," but she'd said he declined to come up from Washington to be with her after Fred asked for a divorce. Elson even grasped the Super Bowl's "gotcha" potential. The kids watched the first half on TV at Fred's; Ally wanted them to come home at halftime. Was her motive "punitive toward [Fred]," Elson wondered, "or simply consistent with her stated belief that the children's bedtime should not be changed?" This was "difficult to determine," he wrote, but "she weakened the this [sic] latter argument by suddenly adding, 'Maybe I would've wanted to watch the second half with them myself,' even though she admittedly had never had an interest in the Super Bowl."

More troublesome are Elson's inferences about family members' character and motives—inferences he characterized as "Clinical Impressions." He wrote, for example, that Raymond "demonstrated real precocity" and "dazzling insights." But he discounted Raymond's preference (to move away with Mom) on the ground that the sixteen-year-old's "ideas about the family" were the product of "longstanding [*sic*], simmering resentments." Raymond, he said, "tended to use his intelligence more for the purpose of shoring up an argument than engaging in fair-minded analysis." Moreover, Raymond was "perceived by others as odd" (Elson didn't say who the "others" were) because his "greatest passions tend to be anchored in a world of rarified, intellectual content." I'm stumped as to what this means (Is what Hannah Arendt called the "life of the mind" odd?), but it's hardly complementary. Nor was Elson complementary of Raymond's response to Fred's following him with a camcorder. Raymond called this a "Gestapo" tactic; Elson characterized this as an "analogy" that "miss[ed] the point." Maybe so, but is this for a psychologist to say? I suspect most people would sympathize with a sixteen-year-old's unhappiness about being tailed by Dad with a video camera. Elson's complaint seems to be that that Raymond's response wasn't "rarified" and "intellectual" enough.

Elson also wielded psychoanalytic language with a serrated edge to support his moral impressions, impressions that influenced his rejection of Ally's plan to move. He dismissed Jack's hostility toward his dad as the product of Ally's having "projected her own sense of feeling powerless and victimized" onto Jack. Jack's resistance to spending time with his father was, in other words, her fault. And Raymond's anger over Fred's abandonment of his mother was the product of his "preoccup[ation] with issues of fairness, both because of his character style and the simple fact that he is an adolescent." Being Mom's "protector," Elson wrote, "allows other unconscious gratifications, such as his supplanting [his dad] as the alpha male within the family."

Nor was Elson cautious when it came to judgments about the lives and opportunities Ally and Fred envisioned for their children. His "clinical" case against Ally's plan to leave New Jersey included this offering of insight and innuendo: "[Ally]'s present interest in a more cosmopolitan experience for the children ignores the arguments that people just as enthusiastically make on behalf of suburbs. While it is understandable that a single or divorced adult might prefer a city, considering all it has to offer, it is hard to dismiss suburbs as a reasonable setting for children, since couples who move from cities to suburbs typically do so for the sake of their children."

Elson issued other verdicts, unconnected to his expertise, about the best balance between parenting and career and about the children's educational opportunities.

His unrestrained approach to the rendering of judgments had toxic effects. It infuriated Ally and Raymond, who mobilized for war, as did Fred. Lawyers hurled charges. The parties took these personally. A Balkan cycle of rage and response ensued. Eventually Ally prevailed in court, winning permission to move to the Washington area, which she did with the two boys. Ana chose to remain in New Jersey with her father. Raymond thrived, putting his violent outbursts behind and focusing on his studies. He was accepted into a prestigious college, where he excelled.

But the shattered relationships were never repaired. When I met with Raymond in September 2010 for an interview, he described his dad as "evil," "abusive," and "corrupt." "He did terrible things," Raymond said. "He's done far too much for me to have a normal relationship and forget about what happened." In the midst of our conversation, his father phoned. His dad called often, Raymond told me, tapping the "ignore" key. Just small talk, Raymond explained—trivial stuff, meant to get under his skin. "I see my father because that's the only chance I get to see my sister and the only chance I get to see my dog. But I decided this summer that I'm not going to do it anymore."

Hot Buttons

Doctors are moral arbiters on the law's behalf in an expanding range of other realms. The legal battle over "partial birth" abortion, for example, devolved into an argument over whether the procedure is "medically necessary," a question without a scientific answer. Pro-life activists seized on a gruesome truth about some late-term abortions: a fetus that grows beyond a certain point can't be taken safely from a woman's womb without first breaking it into parts. Abortion specialists typically do so inside the womb, killing the fetus in the process, then removing the body parts. But both surgical tools and bony fetal fragments can wound the uterus, or so some doctors have warned; thus a few took up the practice of pulling the living fetus into the birth canal before breaking it apart. Hence the term "partial birth," invented by abortion foes intent on underscoring the killing.

Pro-choice activists claim the practice is "medically necessary" in some cases because it's less risky than breaking up the fetus inside the womb. Pro-lifers insist this isn't the case and that dismembering a living fetus outside the womb is too abhorrent to be accepted as "medically necessary." Both sides mustered gynecologists to testify, in court and to Congress, on the question of medical need. But no scientific studies have assessed the difference in risk (if any) between the two approaches. And the question of whether dismemberment outside the womb is too gruesome to be "medically necessary" (whether or not it's less risky) is a matter of morals and culture, not clinical expertise.

Yet in 1998, a federal district court concluded that a Nebraska law banning "partial birth" abortion violated the U.S. Constitution because, according to clinical experts, the procedure is at times "medically necessary."[44] The court based its ruling on testimony to this effect from a parade of pro-choice gynecologists. Two years later, the Supreme Court affirmed.[45] Writing for the majority, Justice Stephen Breyer conceded the "absence of controlled medical studies" but said the district judge's findings of fact, based on expert testimony, were entitled to deference. Breyer strained awkwardly to transmute the scientific uncertainty and dueling clinical claims into a story about the dangers of Nebraska's ban. "[T]he uncertainty," he wrote, "means a significant likelihood that those who believe that [the "partial birth" procedure] is a safer abortion method in certain circumstances may turn out to be right." Perhaps, but they could just as well turn out to be wrong.

Progressives celebrated a victory for sound medical judgment over anti-abortion politics. They had indeed won a victory: Pro-choice gynecologists' moral preferences, cast as medical knowledge, had become constitutional law. Three years later, in 2003, pro-lifers ventured a legislative reprise. Congress passed its own law banning "partial birth" abortion.[46] Mindful of the Nebraska law's fate—including the justices' deference to the district court's medical necessity finding—Congress included a "finding" that "partial birth" abortion is "never medically necessary."[47] This was enough to swing the constitutional question the other way; in 2007, the justices upheld the federal ban, deferring to Congress's medical necessity finding.[48] This time, it was the pro-choice side's turn for ire. The court had allowed Congress to settle a matter that was for doctors to decide, or so many abortion rights advocates said.

But the congressional "finding" that aroused pro-choice ire settled a moral question, not a technical one. Within constitutional law's constraints, public morals are fair game for legislators. Doctors, no less than other citizens, deserve their say. But they overreach by miscasting their moral preferences as products of their expertise. Justice Breyer's opinion for the court in the Nebraska "partial birth" abortion case turned such overreach into law.

When "hot-button" cultural and moral questions become legal disputes, the temptation to turn to medical expertise to resolve them is strong. It's a gambit litigants often try and courts often endorse, since judges are reluctant to be seen as supplying their own answers to moral controversies. And too often, doctors enthusiastically go along, when they ought to refrain from using their credentials as subterfuge for their cultural and moral preferences. They'll be asked to do so increasingly in the future as medicine's ability to explain behavior grows. Should the law treat gay and lesbian sexual desire as biologically fixed (as law treats race) or a matter of personal choice? And what about drinking, smoking, or eating fatty fast foods: Are these individual choices, or should brewers, growers, and those who peddle these products be held legally responsible for the deaths and disability they cause?

Pills for Thinking and Forgetting

And how about performance-enhancing drugs? By broad consensus, Barry Bonds, Roger Clemens, and the other superstars of baseball's Steroids Era were cheaters: Doctors haven't decreed a "steroid deficiency disorder" for players who aspire to extraordinary power-hitting or pitching. But what about students, scientists and scholars, and corporate risers who sharpen their mental edge with medicines? ADHD and other diagnostic categories empower doctors to prescribe performance boosts and require schools and employers to permit them. At fiercely competitive high schools and colleges, there's a street trade in stimulants like Ritalin and Provigil that rivals the market for recreational drugs. And these drugs are crude compared to the possibilities that loom. Our emerging understanding of the molecular basis of learning and memory is likely to lead to chemicals that sculpt both, rather than just increasing brain arousal.[49]

Proponents of what some call cosmetic neurology say drugs that enhance the mind should be available to all who wish to take them.[50] But we're nowhere near to allowing this. Among the moral qualms at play (beyond the health risks) are concerns about fair competition, zero-sum rivalry (think sixteen-year-olds drugging themselves to do better on the SAT), loss of connection between striving and accomplishment, and inequality of opportunity between pharmaceutical haves and have-nots. The main advantage claimed is excellence, or its pursuit. Cognitive scientist Martha Farah, a leading proponent, rejects the comparison to baseball's steroidal sluggers. Their accomplishments were zero-sum, she argues—measurable only through comparisons to each other—but the strivings of scientists, scholars, artists, and entrepreneurs yield advances for humankind.

Today, physicians draw and police the lines between lawful and clandestine use of drugs that boost performance in school and the workplace. They do so collectively, by creating diagnostic categories that the law treats as license for taking mind-enhancing medicines. And they do so case by case, by deciding whether their patients fit within these categories' fuzzy boundaries. That these boundaries give doctors broad discretion is illustrated by the criteria for ADHD. They're a list of foibles that plenty of us possess, including distractibility, forgetfulness, failure to finish chores, inattention to detail, and "dislike" for "sustained mental effort." If your doctor checks six of nine boxes, you're eligible for this diagnosis,[51] so long as she's willing to say that you've had these shortcomings for six months and that they're "maladaptive." Since, of course, they're "maladaptive" (almost by definition, they lead people to fall short of their own goals or others' expectations), diagnosis is a judgment call—a matter of degree.[52]

As our biological understanding of the brain deepens, the scope of medicine's line-drawing and policing power over performance enhancement will expand. Drugs that sharpen reasoning or remembering are likely to inspire new diagnostic categories, contoured to govern their use. Another life-transforming possibility, now within our reach, is intervention to block the chemical pathways by which long-term memory is laid down. Imagine—no, anticipate (the basic science has been done[53])—drugs that, by blocking these pathways, keep painful memories from forming. Should this be seen as a clinical breakthrough—prevention for everything from posttraumatic stress disorder to bitter memories from a night of intimacy gone sour? Or does memory of the painful past teach us ennobling lessons and permit accountability, to the point that pills for forgetting pose quandaries that merit limits on their use?

I'm inclined to think, for example, that a victim of rape should be able to take the pills if she wants to, but what about her ability to testify to the critical details that convict the rapist? Or what about the terrified soldier who fires wildly at a sniper and kills a four-year-old? Should he take the pills as prophylaxis against agonizing remorse, or should the idea of sending troops into combat with a promise of drug-induced psychic impunity alarm us? Through the diagnostic categories they draw up, as well as their case-by-case clinical judgments, physicians will have much to say about the lines between lawful and illicit use of medicines that expand our capabilities and lessen our vulnerabilities. But the moral stakes are too high to tolerate a medical monopoly over the drawing of these lines. Core questions of fairness and equity, merit, personal accountability, and character are at issue. In a democratic society, these are questions for the lay public and their elected representatives. And when these questions reach the courts under cover of clinical diagnosis, judges should push them out into the open rather than deferring to doctors' answers.

Prescribing for the Law's Purposes

Not only do doctors act as moral arbiters on the law's behalf; they intervene biologically to serve the law's purposes. Physicians kill condemned prisoners with drug cocktails and "chemically castrate" convicted sex offenders. In Saudi Arabia and Iran, they've amputated limbs and removed eyes when ordered to do so by courts that follow Sharia law.[54] Sally Johnson's forced medication of Russell Weston was an instance of court-ordered treatment to restore competence, something doctors have proven willing to do even on death row, when therapeutic "success" means execution.

Physicians who do these things claim humanistic cover. Prescribing lethal drugs on death row, then overseeing their injection, averts end-of-life agony from other methods of killing, they say.[55] Chemical castration (treating offenders with drugs that suppress sex drive by blocking the action of male steroids) allows early, safe release of offenders from prison[56]—indeed, statutes in several states condition parole on consent to such treatment. Enlisting surgeons to perform punitive amputations avoids barbarism (and deadly infections). And, as Johnson argues, medication to restore competence relieves terrifying symptoms and empowers prisoners to participate in decisions about their own lives.

But as the Weston case underscores, doctors who do these things reinforce the legitimacy of the legal regimes they serve. The claim that doing these things is humane—even compatible with Hippocratic ideals—assumes the inevitability of the punitive killing, amputation, or other practices that the doctors are "humanizing." As was the case for the CIA physicians who medicalized waterboarding, there's some bootstrapping going on. Medical involvement helps to make these practices acceptable. If a killer is to be executed or a thief's hand is to be cut off, clinical technique is surely less brutal than the firing squad or the ax. But that's hardly the same as saying that what these doctors do to their "patients"—ranging from the disagreeable to the lethal—is consistent with the Hippocratic Oath.

The Oath in the Courts

Judges have responded to conflict between Hippocratic ideals and the law's expectations with an admixture of avoidance and confusion. To be sure, a few courts have held that Hippocratic duty comes first. A notable example was the Louisiana high court's rejection of that state's bid to medicate Michael Perry, a schizophrenic who murdered his mother and father, refused to plead insanity and was convicted and sentenced to die.[57] His postconviction craziness prompted a psychiatric assessment, which led to a finding that he wasn't competent for execution. Prosecutors prevailed upon the trial court to order involuntary treatment. But Louisiana's supreme court held in 1992 that forcible medication to make a condemned inmate competent for execution was unconstitutionally cruel because it breached medical ethics.[58] It couldn't possibly be in the prisoner's "best medical interest" since clinical success would cause his death. Invoking the Hippocratic Oath, the court said the state's "medicate-to-execute" scheme was punishment, not therapy—cruel and degrading because it denied Perry the dignity afforded by the Oath's promise of benevolence.

In an almost identical case a year later, South Carolina's supreme court took the same position.[59] But in 2003, in yet another case involving chemical restoration of competence on death row, the more influential Eighth Circuit Court of Appeals rejected the approach taken in Louisiana and South Carolina.[60] The Eighth Circuit said the prospect of execution wasn't relevant to the condemned's "best medical interest" since his conviction and sentencing extinguished his "due process interests in life and liberty." The patient had no right to live; thus his doctor should disregard the deadly effect of therapeutic success.

That this view disregarded the doctor's Hippocratic pledge to stand by his patient wasn't lost on the four dissenting judges, who warned that the ruling would "forc[e] the medical community to practice in a manner contrary to its ethical standards." Like the Louisiana supreme court, these judges invoked the Oath. They also pointed to the U.S. Supreme Court's past recognition of medicine's "integrity" as a factor in constitutional interpretation. Six years earlier, in *Washington v. Glucksberg,* the justices had upheld a ban on physician-assisted suicide.[61] Among the justifications they offered for allowing this intrusion into personal choice was the state's "interest in protecting the integrity and ethics of the medical profession." Permitting doctors to help people kill themselves, the court cautioned, could "undermine the trust that is essential to the doctor patient relationship by blurring the time honored line between healing and harming."

The Eighth Circuit dissenters chided their colleagues for ignoring this concern in the capital punishment context. But the Supreme Court allowed the Eighth Circuit's restoration-of-competence ruling to stand.[62] The ruling, a rare *en banc* judgment (i.e., a decision by the entire court as opposed to the usual three-judge panel), is widely seen as an authoritative statement that it's permissible to tell doctors to treat the condemned so the state can kill them.

Four months after the Eighth Circuit issued its ruling, the Supreme Court finally spoke to the question presented when Russell Weston refused treatment: whether the government could forcibly medicate a prisoner solely to make him competent to stand trial.[63] Dangerousness, this time, wasn't an issue. The defendant, Charles Sell, a dentist and right-wing activist with beliefs that bordered on the paranoid—and, in prison doctors' view, crossed the border—was charged with Medicare fraud. The justices produced a convoluted opinion that, in theory, allowed the authorities to medicate Sell but, in practice, put up enough obstacles to make doing so exceedingly difficult.[64] Writing for the majority, Justice Breyer predicted that involuntary medication to restore trial competence would be "rare." But he avoided any mention of Hippocratic ideals. He cast the doctors who give the drugs as state functionaries, with no duty of fidelity to their patients.

Five years later, the court took a sharply different approach to the question of whether Hippocratic fidelity counted on death row. Inmates awaiting execution in several states had challenged the constitutionality of lethal injection, claiming that the usual procedure constitutes "cruel and unusual punishment." The standard approach kills in three steps—painlessly if all goes well. First, the executioner administers a barbiturate intravenously; the purpose of this drug is to put the prisoner to sleep for what comes next. Then—here's the dicey part—the executioner injects a synthetic version of curare, a poison once used by South American hunters to kill animals by paralyzing their respiratory muscles. This drug is given mostly as a matter of decorum (to prevent unsightly gasping and twitching); death results from the third step, an injection of potassium chloride to stop the heart. Lawyers for condemned inmates claimed that, too often, all did *not* go well. Too small a dose of the barbiturate, they said, left some prisoners alert and aware for the terror and agony of steps 2 and 3.

Putting doctors in the execution chamber to ensure an adequate dose would solve this problem, just as medicating the condemned to make them competent clears the last legal obstacle to carrying out the sentence. But when the challenge to the three-step procedure reached the Supreme Court, the justices said physician assistance wasn't an option because professional ethics didn't permit it.[65] In a concurring opinion, Justice Samuel Alito said "modification of a lethal injection protocol cannot be regarded as 'feasible' . . . if the modification would require participation . . . by persons whose professional ethics rules or traditions impede their participation."[66] He noted that "the ethics rules of medical professionals—for reasons that I certainly do not question here—prohibit their participation."

On this basis, the court said there wasn't a "feasible" way to reduce the risk of suffering from the three-step method. Cynics might suggest that the justices (and courts more generally) use clinical ethics as a tool to support conclusions they've already reached on other grounds. It's clear that the court invoked medical ethics artfully, to turn back a challenge to capital punishment's constitutional survival. Death-penalty opponents had hoped to end lethal injection by making medical participation legally necessary. Doctors, they figured, would say no, putting a stop to state killing.[67] By deferring to the profession's position, then finding that the three-step method, *sans* physicians, didn't pose "substantial risk" of suffering, the court averted this double bind, allowing executions to continue. Likewise, the justices had decided for other reasons to uphold Washington State's ban on assisted suicide[68]; thus their reference to "the integrity and ethics of the medical profession" may have been a mere add-on.

Courts' willingness to count Hippocratic fidelity in other contexts has been spotty. The privacy of what patients tell their doctors rarely receives protection when it stands in the way of the law's other purposes. Nor need doctors worry about legal sanctions when they judge their patients harshly, then share such judgments with the courts. Ally encountered this in wounding fashion when custody evaluators and a lawyer appointed by the court to make custody recommendations contacted the therapists she and her family had seen.[69] A psychologist who had worked with Ally and Fred told the lawyer Ally was "malignant," an observation the lawyer quoted in her report to the court. According to the same report, Jack's psychiatrist characterized Ally as "out of touch," "clueless," "passive aggressive," and "brutal"—and called Jack "jealous." And the psychologist Ally and Fred consulted for Raymond's attention and anger problems said Ally had turned her sons against Fred as a way of coping with her insecurities.

Not only do the courts shield clinical caregivers from legal sanctions for such breaches of fidelity; the law often mandates this sort of betrayal. Doctors have no choice but to share their patients' clinical histories and other intimate life details with custody evaluators. In some jurisdictions, patients must first "consent" to such revelation. But since the threat of losing one's children looms over the process, refusal to cooperate with an evaluator by giving this consent can hardly be called voluntary. The circumstances are similar for other high-stakes forensic inquiries—into competence, criminal responsibility, and disability. What you tell your internist, gynecologist, or psychotherapist can be used against you in legal proceedings down the line. How many Americans are stunned each year by such betrayals of faith isn't known. But I suspect the number is quite high, in the hundreds of thousands or more, due to the chasm between people's expectations of Hippocratic fidelity and the legal system's lack of regard for it.

Doctors who perform assessments for the law's purposes claim immunity from the complaint that they're violating Hippocratic obligation. Their duty is to the court or the client, they contend, and the people they evaluate shouldn't be mistaken for patients. Some have gone so far as to say they don't act as doctors, the same argument pressed by the Pentagon in the interrogation context. "[T]he forensic psychiatrist in truth does not act as a physician," one of the field's most influential commentators, Paul Appelbaum, wrote in 1990.[70] In an article that many forensic practitioners regard as seminal, Appelbaum said a "different—nonmedical—role with its own ethical values is involved." "Truth," in the interest of "justice," is the forensic evaluator's purpose, he opined. "Doing harm" isn't cause for "anguish," but failure to do one's best "in the difficult quest for truth" is.

I have trouble understanding Appelbaum's alternative to medical ethics. How is an ethic of "truth" to guide the moral judgments that animate medical opinions on such matters as competence, criminal responsibility, and child custody? Are doctors' opinions supposed to be stand-ins for *society's* moral preferences? Or do doctors have some sort of special moral expertise, a proposition of which I've been skeptical throughout this book? Appelbaum's claim that forensic evaluators don't act as physicians, though, is plainly wrong. Not only do they use their clinical skills and specialized knowledge to perform assessments (just as CIA and military doctors drew on their clinical know-how to design interrogations); they gain courtroom credibility from medicine's scientific and humanistic aura.

Beyond that, they trade on their identity as clinical caregivers in the minds of the men and women they assess. And if they're good at what they do, they win these people's trust. To be sure, forensic evaluators make a practice of saying at the outset that they're not serving in a therapeutic role—that instead, they're rendering opinions for courts or others—and that these opinions could go against those being evaluated. But then, a process of seduction begins. Especially in psychiatry and psychology, but also in neurology, occupational medicine, and other fields that play forensic roles, good clinical assessment requires empathic connection—the caring voice, knowing smiles, and willingness to listen that inspire trust. The best clinicians are often naturals: Recall Sally Johnson's observation that she didn't choose psychiatry so much as psychiatry found her, as people sought her out to tell her about their lives. But this gift can be taught. Good clinical training aims to do so. And clinicians can tap people's predispositions to trust them—predispositions born of faith in medicine as a benevolent endeavor. Boilerplate disclosure at the beginning of an interview—caveats about courtroom use and lack of clinical confidentiality—doesn't dispel these predispositions or forestall the feelings of connection that a good clinician encourages. Nor is dissolution of trust the forensic evaluator's goal; to the contrary, its preservation is vital to his or her craft.

For evaluators sensitive to the paradox inherent in nurturing people's trust, then issuing judgments that betray it, Appelbaum's assurance that "doing harm" isn't cause for "anguish" rings hollow. Anguish, or, at least, unease, is a morally authentic response to the poor fit between the Hippocratic promise of fidelity and what forensic practitioners do. This unease ought to energize efforts to limit what the law asks of them. And it should inspire them to set their own limits on the services they provide. Moral overreach of the sort I've described should be beyond this pale. So should gate-keeping roles (such as opining on competence to be executed) that could have a devastating impact on the people these practitioners assess. As even the Supreme Court has recognized, albeit inconsistently, medicine's identity and credibility as a compassionate endeavor rest on society's willingness to abide by such limits. Unease, even anguish, over our incompatible public and intimate expectations of medicine can mobilize our efforts to mediate between them.

chapter ten

conclusion

moving beyond the myth

Dr. Kapil

“Dad, what are you going to do if the prisoner isn't dead?” The question taunted Balvir Kapil. A dozen times, he'd done his duty. Each time, he'd gotten lucky. A corrections officer turned a key, starting the machines. Then another officer pressed a button, setting off a sequence of power surges. High and low voltages alternated over a period of three minutes. Each surge coursed through the body of the condemned, across sponge-covered, saline-soaked metal contact points fixed to his scalp and leg. After a wait of a few minutes more, Dr. Kapil approached the prisoner to perform a brief examination. He looked and listened for signs of life—a few gasps or a heartbeat. Seeing and hearing nothing, he pronounced death—and walked away relieved.

When all goes well, there's smoke and steam where skin and metal meet. The body jerks, spasms, then slumps into the straight-backed wooden chair. To make death highly likely, redundancy is designed in. High voltage stops the heart. Low voltage alters its rhythms in ways that usually kill. But electrical killing is an art, not a science. Hearts paused by high voltage can resume beating when the current ebbs. And high voltage can convert an erratic rhythm (induced by a low-voltage surge) to a normal heartbeat, a fact physicians use to save lives. Other problems can arise—equipment failures and bad connections.

Once, while Dr. Kapil was on vacation, another physician subbed for him at an execution. Prison officials strapped the condemned into the chair, covered his face with the ritual leather mask, and delivered the prescribed voltage. The doctor approached the man, listened with a stethoscope, and told the assembled witnesses, "He has not expired." The nightmare scenario pressed by Kapil's son Vikram, who'd started law school around the time his father began to attend executions, was playing out.

Medical ethics has a clear answer to the question of what a doctor should do in this situation. He or she should take emergency measures—pulmonary resuscitation if the prisoner isn't breathing, full-fledged CPR if his heart stops—going all-out to save the prisoner's life. That's the position professional societies and ethics commentators have taken almost without exception. The Commonwealth of Virginia also had a clear answer. The physician should inform the executioners that their work wasn't yet done, then step aside to let them finish.

When I spoke with Vikram Kapil recently,[1] he recalled being relentless with his father on this point:

> We argued about that. "Dad, what are you going to do if the prisoner isn't dead? You're going to have to revive him. And then they're going to electrocute him again." . . . "Well," he said, "the law has to be followed." And I said, "So you're going to go in and revive him and they're going to electrocute him again?" And he said, "Well, that's not right."

So Vikram's father came to the conclusion that letting the executioners have another go was the wrong thing to do. But he'd signed on to this work—to attending executions, pronouncing death, and, if necessary, allowing prison officers to try again. In 1990, after a decade as a prison doctor, he'd become chief physician at Virginia's Department of Corrections. "He knew, at the time he applied for the job, that attending executions was part of the job," Vikram told me. So he continued to do so as death sentences became more frequent, suppressing his "what if" worries even after his substitute was forced to face the question. That his colleague had resolved the matter by stepping aside—by doing nothing to help the survivor (whom the executioners killed on their next try)—made defiance of the commonwealth's expectations seem even harder.

I knew none of this in March 1994, when a National Public Radio producer asked me to come on to *All Things Considered* to talk about a report I'd coauthored on medical participation in executions. Figuring that I'd be less interesting than a doctor who actually took part, I suggested she find one. Virginia seemed a likely place to look.[2] That's how she discovered Dr. Kapil. Within a few days, Dr. Kapil and I were in an NPR studio to tape a segment that host Daniel Zwerdling would later call "a little bit astonishing."[3] An early hint came when Zwerdling asked what happens when the executioners switch off the current:

> DR. KAPIL: They wait about three, four—three or four minutes. And then the officer comes and asks me to enter the chamber.
>
> ZWERDLING: And then?
>
> DR. KAPIL: Then I examine the patient and pronounce death. I turn to the warden and I say, "This man has expired."
>
> ZWERDLING: It's interesting that you use the word "patient."[4]

Zwerdling brought up the Hippocratic Oath. Kapil insisted he hadn't violated it. Then Zwerdling asked about the messy execution that Kapil, by happenstance, had missed:

> ZWERDLING: Had you been there, you would have had to make that decision, whether the man was dead or not, and if he weren't, what would you have done?
>
> DR. KAPIL: Well, I agree with you that this is possible, but I think the probability of this happening is—approaches zero.[5]

Deftly, Zwerdling let this evasion stand for a moment, then came at the question from another direction:

ZWERDLING: According to my schedule, your corrections department is going to execute somebody in a few weeks—supposing they call you a few minutes after they think he's died, and supposing you find that his heart is beating. What will you do?

DR. KAPIL: Well, that is a dilemma. . . .

ZWERDLING: So there is something about participating around these executions that does seem to discomfort you.

DR. KAPIL: There are troubling questions, I have to admit that.

ZWERDLING: When you're alone at night, and you're drinking a cup of tea, and you start to think about the things that trouble you, what does trouble you about this?

DR. KAPIL: This very thing that you mentioned, the rare probability that it may not have been successful. Then I would be torn between my duty to start resuscitation and then my medical duty as a professional, and my other duty which is to turn around and tell the warden to give additional—take additional measures.[6]

The segment aired nationwide on April 3. A few days later, Dr. Kapil told a local reporter that he was "leaning" toward the position that pronouncing death at executions was unethical.[7] The following week, the *Washington Post* reported that Kapil planned to go "on holiday" for future executions. The next, the case Zwerdling had mentioned, loomed later in the month—a high-profile affair involving the first-ever death sentence based on a DNA match. The details of the crimes were gruesome, and Governor George Allen, thinking himself presidential timber, was intent on showing relentlessness in carrying out the jury's will.

Newspapers around the country carried the story of Kapil's ethical shudder, angering the governor and the law-and-order men around him. Allen's staff sent word to Kapil that he'd be removed from his post unless he continued to pronounce.[8] American Medical Association officials told Kapil he'd have their public support if he refused and was fired. Anti–death-penalty activists warmed to the prospect of having a martyr of sorts around whom to make their case. But Kapil would have none of this. "He was a company man," his son told me. "He had an Indian attitude—let's take care of this quietly. . . . He knew what pressures everyone was under." And, said Vikram, "he was trying to please everyone."

But trying to please everyone had its costs. Six years earlier, at age fifty-four, Kapil had suffered a small stroke. By the beginning of 1994, months before his appearance on NPR, he'd developed cardiac symptoms, including difficulty breathing when he walked briskly. Through the spring, the pressure mounted. His conviction deepened that as a doctor, he had no place in the execution chamber. And he dreaded what might happen to his professional reputation if he went back in. But he feared losing his job—its health and retirement benefits, comfortable salary, and considerable cachet. And he was intent on avoiding a public confrontation.

Kapil finessed the next execution, on April 27, by taking a vacation day. The private physician who pronounced death in his stead declared, "The AMA is not great God almighty." Going on holiday, though, was hardly a long-term solution. And his efforts to negotiate a behind-the-scenes resolution seemed to be going nowhere. As the pressures tightened, his health worsened. "The stress of the situation was playing on him," his son recalled. By the summer, merely taking a few steps was making him short of breath. Meanwhile, more executions loomed.

On August 14, NPR's Daniel Zwerdling revisited the story he'd helped to create. Zwerdling brought Kapil back on air to talk about his change of mind. Kapil announced that he'd made a deal with the state to keep his job without pronouncing death. "State law says that it has to be a physician, not the chief physician," he said. Other doctors were willing. He was, as Zwerdling put it, "off the hook." But by August, Kapil's own doctors were recommending bypass surgery. The operation was scheduled for September, just after the birth of his first grandchild. From the start, his surgeons encountered the unexpected. Complications developed, then cascaded disastrously. He died in the operating room, leaving behind his widow, four children, and Vikram's newborn daughter.

What Our Doctors Owe Us

We hold warring ideas about what our doctors owe us. Dr. Kapil and his family became collateral damage in this conflict. Our failure to clarify the limits on medicine's public role left him without legal and ethical safe haven. We expect commitment, without compromise, to our needs as individuals. Yet we ask medicine to serve myriad social purposes, from health care cost containment to criminal justice, national security, and support for our common values. We call upon doctors not only to affirm and enforce these values but to choose between them when they contradict. And often we ask doctors to shield these choices from our gaze so we can stay in denial about painful compromises. Increasingly, moreover, we marshal medical technologies to pursue public objectives, such as national security and criminal punishment. And increasingly, we're putting medicine's credibility as a caring endeavor at risk by pushing doctors to break faith with their Hippocratic pledge of fidelity to patients.

Until the time of Hippocrates, medicine's intimate and public purposes weren't at odds. In the ancient cosmologies that have come down to us through religious texts, historical accounts, and archeological inquiry, illness was a matter of being out of sorts with the divine. Clear distinctions weren't drawn between citizens' obligations to the gods, the state, and each other. Doctors (and the priests who preceded them) healed by bringing their patients' bodies and minds into harmony with divine—and social and cultural—expectations. Healing and public purposes were thus paired, or at least closely tied. Then the Hippocratics introduced something radical: the claim that sickness is material and secular. Illness, they held, isn't an expression of the gods' wrath, or society's; thus, the work of healing is something apart from state and social purposes. Patients' needs and interests, therefore, often diverge from public ends. The Hippocratic promise of fidelity to patients follows from this divergence. It assures the sick that they can count on doctors to put their needs, hopes, and fears first.

Medicine's public roles have expanded enormously since the Hippocratics made this revolutionary advance. The profession's scientific foundations, technical capabilities, and cultural authority have made it a potent force in

our civil and social lives. Health care's sheer cost accounts for much of medicine's public import. Spending is soaring toward 20 percent of America's
economy, a milestone we'll pass before this decade is out. The health reform legislation enacted in 2010 did nothing to alter the combustible mix
of third-party payment and technological advance that's the main driver of
medical costs.[9] Longer-term projections call for health spending to reach 40
percent of gross domestic product by mid-century. We're not willing to foot
this bill, either as consumers or as taxpayers. But neither are we willing to
forgo the therapeutic possibilities this spending promises.

So we put our doctors in the middle. We expect them to provide care
whenever potential benefits outweigh risks, yet we demand that they set limits. It's easy to vilify Dr. Jose Arevelo, the health plan medical director who
said no to Carrie Emard's endometriosis surgery, for withholding a treatment
that could spare her a lifetime of pain. But health plans must keep to bud-
gets that are constrained by their customers' willingness to pay for coverage.
Dr. Arevelo had to make do within this budget; otherwise, Carrie's HMO
couldn't remain a going concern. And it's easy to condemn Dr. Lori Pegram for endangering Cynthia Herdrich's life by delaying her ultrasound for
a week, but the Carle Clinic, likewise, had to stay within budget to survive.
Both health plans employed financial rewards to coax doctors to practice
cheaply. This strategy suborns doctors to violate their Hippocratic vow of
fidelity, but it's a powerful tool for limiting medical spending.

More crudely, Yanira Montanez's doctors at two inner-city emergency
rooms cut corners amid scarce resources, with catastrophic results. A Philadelphia jury understandably found them negligent; they overlooked key physical findings and didn't order follow-up lab studies to assess life-endangering
risks. But they worked within tight constraints imposed on them by voters and
public officials, who have proven unwilling to provide the resources needed to
bring health services for the poor up to par with care for the well off.

The doctors in these cases adjusted what they did on behalf of their
patients to fit the available means. Soaring costs and rising imbalance between clinical resources and therapeutic possibilities will require ever-greater
adjustment of this sort. But the Hippocratic Myth doesn't countenance such

accommodation. The Myth calls on clinicians to give their all to each patient, without regard for society's constraints. The Myth thus keeps doctors from admitting the need for accommodation. Beyond that, it reinforces the public's expectation that doctors can somehow provide all care that yields net benefit—an expectation that has, so far, made serious political discussion of medical cost containment impossible.

Medicine also has a growing role as arbiter and enforcer of public morality. Clinical diagnosis incorporates beliefs about the scope of personal responsibility, the levels of distress people should be expected to endure, and the divide between what we should accept and seek to change about the human condition. Diagnosis imports these beliefs, unexamined, into our politics, culture, and law. Posttraumatic stress disorder (PTSD) illustrates this point: Embedded premises about the suffering soldiers and others should abide shape both its formal definition and the judgments of clinicians in individual cases. Debates over whether obesity, short stature, and myriad other physical and mental states constitute diseases reflect underlying conflicts among cultural and moral premises. Diagnosis often forgives, since it depicts our shortcomings as biologically determined. But it sometimes accuses, by pointing a finger at those (e.g., tobacco growers and sellers of fatty foods) who exploit our biological vulnerabilities.

Medicine's role as arbiter of public morals extends beyond clinical diagnosis. Child custody, criminal culpability, and legal competency have become the province of physicians and psychologists. Doctors opine on whether same-sex desire is chosen or biologically determined, when life begins and ends, and when disability merits support from the public dole. Courts, pundits, and politicians welcome this opinion-giving. It takes judges off the hook for hard decisions, and it lends rhetorical backing to ideological preconceptions. More often than not, medicine's scientific aura obscures the underlying moral judgments. The Hippocratic Myth adds a blush of benevolence, encouraging confidence in doctors' answers to contested questions even when these answers don't rest on real expertise.

Medicine's national security role is poised to grow explosively. America's post-9/11 misadventure with interrogation bordering on torture underscores both the attractions and the dangers of putting biomedical science to military use. Not only did psychologists and physicians design and oversee the abuse inflicted on detainees at clandestine CIA centers and elsewhere; these professionals played key roles in justifying it. In the legal memos that made the Bush administration's case, medical oversight lent a sense of precision and constraint. Again, the auras of science and benevolence reassured and misled, sending the message that even waterboarding and physical assaults were designed clinically (in both senses of this word) to extract intelligence while minimizing "medical" risk.

What the Bush administration did to put the pressure on post-9/11 detainees was quite low tech. But the national security possibilities that loom ahead seem more like the stuff of sci-fi. Drugs that block—or boost—the biological mechanisms of human resilience, agents that interfere with formation of traumatic memories, and chemical enhancements of war-fighters' focus and alertness are under development, building on science that's already been done. Diagnostic imaging techniques, including functional magnetic resonance imaging and computerized analysis of electroencephalogram patterns, are being honed as tools for assessing intelligence sources' truthfulness. And a new generation of biological weaponry is emerging—drugs and other technologies designed to interfere in nonlethal fashion with the physiology of hostage-holding terrorists or insurgents hiding amid civilians. Some of these developments could make war-fighting less brutal and more effective. Others could make it more devastating.

In civilian life as well, clinical methods are increasingly being put to nontherapeutic use. Medicalization of executions, athletic performance, and scholastic achievement has set off controversies but continued apace. Executions of the sort Dr. Kapil attended have become rare; lethal injection now prevails. When, in 2008, the Supreme Court rejected the claim that lethal injection constitutes cruel and unusual punishment, the justices reviewed the standard three-drug protocol and noted its near painlessness.[10] They permitted physicians to refuse to assist, a development that bodes well for future efforts by the profession to set limits on its public roles. But the medical science supporting the drugs' use was key to the court's constitutional endorsement.

Pharmacological enhancement of athletic performance is almost universally seen as cheating. Baseball's Steroids Era and cycling's blood-doping scandals undermined these sports' perceived legitimacy. Competitors in these and other sports must now comply with intrusive drug-testing regimens. Doctors who've prescribed banned substances face prosecution. But orthopedic surgeons are collaborating with computer scientists on 3-D "motion capture" methods that boost performance by helping athletes to custom-tailor their running and throwing to their anatomical constraints. Under a shroud of secrecy, the San Francisco Giants are applying this technology to their pitchers' deliveries.[11] (The Giants, according to a *New York Times* account, have refused even to confirm the location of their program, let alone allow outsiders to see it.[12]) That the Giants shocked baseball by winning the 2010 World Series with a team of cast-offs anchored by extraordinary pitching may or may not be related to what their doctors are doing. But it will surely spur interest.

Use of drugs to boost academic performance has gone mainstream. It's routine, under cover of clinical diagnosis, at competitive high schools and colleges. And it's becoming common, even absent diagnosis, thanks to demanding parents and teachers, driven students, and ample street supplies. Doctors draw the boundaries of legitimate cognitive enhancement by settling on diagnostic criteria. But there's mounting pressure to expand these boundaries, both by loosening diagnostic criteria to permit wider "therapeutic" use and by allowing doctors to prescribe enhancers absent a diagnosis.[13]

As this book went to press, an American Academy of Neurology panel had begun work on practice guidelines for prescription of enhancers to the healthy. Drugs already available have been shown to boost learning, memory, and so-called executive functioning (tuning out distractions, suppressing emotional responses, and switching efficiently between tasks) in many people who don't qualify for clinical diagnoses. Agents under development promise to spur the formation of lasting memories by influencing genetic control of protein synthesis. Possibilities farther down the line include drugs that could enable us to manage our moods, bringing forth different states of mind to cope with the varied tasks of life and work.

So long as people can choose whether to take such drugs for performance enhancement purposes, prescribing them can be seen as an extension of patient care. But medicine can't take this path without staking out positions on matters of morality and character.[14] Our beliefs about the meaning of merit and the ties between striving and virtue are challenged by chemical self-improvement. And unless the new biology of self-improvement is made available to all, irrespective of economic standing, use of these agents will amplify social inequity. Moreover, people's "choices" to take these drugs may not always be worthy of deference. Such choice is often the product of intense pressure, resulting from rivalry for fixed stakes. The SAT, high school grades, and admission to Stanford or Yale aren't win-win propositions: it's comparative performance that counts.[15] So if "everyone else is doing it," it may be madness (or seem like it) to say no. It may be better in such circumstances for doctors to say no, to avoid chemical arms races that yield no net benefit.

Between Personal Fidelity and Public Duty

We're nowhere near to squaring our expectations of doctors as caregivers with medicine's myriad public roles. The Hippocratic Myth stands in the way. At a time when medicine commands nearly a fifth of the U.S. economy, we insist that our doctors care for us without regard for cost. With rare exceptions, they reassure us that they do. To admit otherwise—to openly balance costs against benefits—would violate our expectations and the medical profession's sense of itself. So we pursue health care cost control by stealth, inveighing our doctors to say no covertly and offering them financial rewards for doing so. But inevitably, stealth fails us—clandestine cost-awareness becomes the stuff of scandal. Being "quietly and gently hypocritical," as Sara Eisenberg's cardiologist put it, won't work.

It didn't work in Sara's case, and it hasn't worked for our country. The late 1990s backlash against managed care underscored this, and the absurdist rancor over "death panels" and "rationing boards" during the battle over health care reform demonstrated the lingering toxicity of distrust from past hypocrisies exposed. The irony is that when it comes to cost, the 2010 health reform law did so little. Leaving current ways of doing things intact, with minor tweaks, was the political price for expanding medical coverage to 30 million Americans who now lack it.

This price was worth paying in the short run to protect 30 million people from the Darwinian cruelty of lack of access to basic care. But it's not affordable over the long term. We'll need to find ways to control soaring spending without imperiling clinical caregivers' perceived trustworthiness and without setting off a wave of electoral repudiation of the sort that washed over Congress after health reform passed. In this book, I've mapped a path toward doing so. It's a path that promises to slow development of the pricey, high-tech, low-benefit tests and treatments that are the main drivers of medical spending—and to thereby reduce pressure on doctors and insurers to say no to available therapeutic options. But it does involve the explicit setting of limits. It would make cost-benefit trade-off policies increasingly transparent, at a pace that matches Americans' gradual adjustment to the reality that such trade-offs are essential. It would foster clinical guidelines that put these policies into practice, and it would allow economic rewards for physicians who follow them.

But suborning doctors to withhold care covertly deserves no place in any cost-containment strategy that's designed to endure. Reward schemes that allow caregivers to profit through furtive skimping are recipes for popular anger and erosion of trust. Promising patients all "medically necessary" care, then paying doctors in ways that promote stinting on the sly, is a shortsighted alternative to confronting the disconnect between our expectations as patients and our willingness to foot the bill as consumers and taxpayers.

Looking to doctors to resolve matters of public morality under cover of clinical judgment is no less shortsighted. Not only does it usurp the roles of public officials and popular will in democratic governance; it sets the stage for backlash and distrust when clinical cover is blown. "Medical" judgments about personal responsibility, right conduct, and appropriate desire are sooner or later exposed as moral impositions. The popular ire over psychiatry run amok that followed John Hinckley's successful insanity plea is a case in point.

Eventually, I suspect, there'll be a similar backlash against the virtual takeover of child custody litigation by mental health professionals. In the courtroom and the public realm more generally, doctors should refrain from opining as experts on such questions as who should be held criminally accountable, responsible for obesity, or best suited to raise children. They can and should contribute as experts on diagnosis and treatment of impairment, but they shouldn't go beyond what science supports.

When diagnosis and therapy rest on answers to contested questions of public morality, doctors ought to admit this and consider these questions openly. Efforts to set diagnostic criteria and treatment protocols without acknowledging these questions aren't just disingenuous; they're sure to engender mistrust. The American experience with PTSD illustrates this. Successive efforts by leaders in psychiatry and related fields to redefine PTSD have treated the task as a technical matter, disregarding its political content. But moral and cultural politics are at the heart of controversy over PTSD. They've animated conservatives' efforts to narrow the diagnosis and liberals' impassioned resistance. The framers of diagnostic criteria and therapeutic options for PTSD and other politically charged illnesses will need to find ways to involve the lay public in their moral decision-making. At a minimum, proposed diagnostic schemes and treatment protocols should be clear about their moral premises so as to foster discussion and dampen distrust. So should emerging protocols for performance enhancement in the classroom, at the workplace, and on the battlefield.

Use of medical methods for national security, criminal justice, and other state purposes needn't be rejected per se. Absent a clinical relationship, Hippocratic fidelity is beside the point; what matters is that such uses comport with precepts of decency that we hold to in nonclinical contexts. As new technologies emerge, their fit with human rights principles, the laws of war, and social mores will often be subject to dispute, but the role-related ethics of doctor-patient relations shouldn't be at issue.

When there's a clinical relationship, matters are more complicated. It doesn't work, I've argued in this book, to say that the doctor who medicates a prisoner to make him competent for execution isn't acting as a physician and needn't worry about Hippocratic ethics. But it's unreasonable to insist on Hippocratic purity to the point of barring all uses of clinical skill on society's behalf. The challenge—for society, not just for the medical profession—is to negotiate boundaries between acceptable and improper exploitation of clinical relationships for public purposes. Considerations include the import of the social purpose at stake (and the value-added that doctors bring), the implications for trust and trustworthiness in therapeutic relationships, and the strain on doctors' shared identity as caregivers committed to standing by their patients.

Subjective judgments are necessary, and broad input is essential, to mediate wisely between medicine's caregiving responsibilities and its proliferating public roles. It's a myth that medicine is self-governing in ethical matters. The profession crafts and reconceives its ethics in conversation with society's expressions of need. Market forces, political pressures, cultural change, and law's demands nudge medicine's ethics in different directions over time. Hippocratic fidelity is itself an outcome of this interplay. Its contours, I've contended here, have evolved in response to waxing and waning concerns about the fragility of patients' trust.

This evolution, though, can't be taken for granted; nor can the resilience of patients' trust. Medicine's expanding social roles are putting this trust at unprecedented risk. A national discussion is needed about the fit between what we expect from our doctors at the bedside and clinic and what we're increasingly asking them to do in the public realm. The Hippocratic Myth, though, stands in the way. It nurtures the impression that no accommodation is necessary—that we can somehow demand our doctors' undivided devotion (and care without regard for cost) while calling upon them to control medical spending, wage war, and take sides in legal and moral conflicts. The Myth likewise pressures doctors to deny that they compromise patients' interests to serve public purposes, since it holds that doing so is wrong. It thereby stymies discussion of prudent accommodation between medicine's caregiving and social roles.

In so doing, the Myth sets us against ourselves and puts doctors in the crossfire. It's easy to admonish Lori Pegram for taking money to stint on care, Scott Uithol for his role at Abu Ghraib, and Balvir Kapil for becoming a cog in state killing. But as a society, we've asked them to do these things. We've gone through channels. Dr. Pegram went by her HMO's rules, which rewarded her for frugality in a fashion the Supreme Court endorsed. Dr. Uithol followed orders despite his doubts. And Dr. Kapil went by Virginia law, until a mix of embarrassment and conscience led him to say no.

The consequences of failure to move beyond the Myth would be enormous. To stave off long-term fiscal disaster, we'll need to contain soaring health spending. But cost control on the down low won't work. We're too good, as a society, at seeing through our self-deceptions. Until we're able to speak openly about forgoing therapeutic benefits, a possibility the Myth doesn't abide, serious efforts to set limits will fail amid toxic recriminations. And unless we're able to move beyond the Myth, toward forthright consideration of medicine's proliferating moral and political roles, the cloaking of moral propositions in clinical guise will proceed apace, intruding on democratic institutions of governance. The irony is that the Myth has become an *obstacle* to Hippocratic trustworthiness and trust, which can only be sustained by candor about medicine's growing place in the public realm.

notes

Chapter One   Introduction

1. The events I relate here occurred in the spring of 1997, at a nursing and hospice care facility. "Dr. Mara" is a pseudonym.
2. Congressional Budget Office, "The Long-Term Outlook for Health Care Spending," Pub. No. 3085 (2007). www.cbo.gov/ftpdocs/87xx/doc8758/11–13-LT-Health.pdf
3. This premise found expression in non-western traditions. Swearers to an Arabic oath promise: "In all my treatment I will strive so far as lies in my power for the benefit of the patients." The Indian *Oath of Charaka* announces: "Day and night, however thou mayest be engaged, thou shalt endeavor for the relief of patients with all thy heart and soul."
4. See Howard Markel, "'I Swear by Apollo'—On Taking the Hippocratic Oath," *New England Journal of Medicine* 350, no. 20 (May 2008): 2026–2029. The first recorded administration of the oath in a medical school was in 1508 at the University of Wittenberg in Germany; it did not become a standard part of medical school graduation until 1804. Administration of the oath became prominent in North American medical schools only after accounts of Nazi medical atrocities during World War II gave rise to an increased interest in ethics.
5. Clinical psychologists, nurse-practitioners, and other patient-care professionals don't recite the Oath at graduation, but their ethical precepts include this commitment.
6. Plato, *Plato's Phaedrus,* trans. Albert A. Anderson (Millis, MA: Agora Publications, 2009), 71–72. "Both medicine and rhetoric proceed by analyzing nature; one examines the body, and the other examines the soul. They succeed not simply on the basis of tradition and experience—medicine attends to health and strength through the art of providing medication and nutrition, and rhetoric seeks it through the teaching and practice of sound thinking and goodness of the soul."
7. Mark A. Hall et al., "Trust in Physicians and Medical Institutions: What Is It, Can It Be Measured, and Does It Matter?" *Milbank Quarterly* 79, no. 4 (2001): 614. "As an instrumental value, trust is widely believed to be essential to effective therapeutic encounters. It has been hypothesized or shown to affect a host of important behaviors and attitudes, including patients' willingness to seek care, reveal sensitive information, submit to treatment, participate in research, adhere to treatment regimens, remain with a physician, and recommend physician to others. In addition, it may mediate clinical outcomes. Commentators speculate that trust is a key factor in the mind-body interactions that underlie placebo effects, the effectiveness of alternative medicine, and unexplained variations in outcomes from conventional therapies."
8. Roy Porter, *The Greatest Benefit to Mankind: A Medical History of Humanity* (London, UK: Norton, 1997), 367.
9. Ibid.

10. Henry E. Sigerist, "From Bismarck to Beveridge: Developments and Trends in Social Security Legislation," *Journal of Public Health Policy* 20, no. 4 (1999): 474–496, 487.

11. For example, in the United Kingdom, roughly .05 percent of gross domestic product was GDP spent on health care at the beginning of the twentieth century. www.ukpublicspending.co.uk/spending_brief.php

12. *R. v. M'Naughten,* 8 Eng. Rep. 718 (H.L. 1843).

13. *State v. Pike,* 49 N.H. 399, 441–442 (1869). "If he does know the act to be wrong, he is equally irresponsible whether his will is overcome, and his hand used, by the irresistible power of his own mental disease, or by the irresistible power of another person. When disease is the propelling, uncontrollable power, the man is as innocent as the weapon,— the mental and moral elements are as guiltless as the material."

14. See *M'Naughten,* supra n. 12.

Chapter Two   Cutting Costs and Keeping Faith

1. Telephone interview with Carrie Emard, September 2008.

2. *Endometrium* is the medical term for the tissue that lines the uterus—highly-vascularized tissue that nourishes the early embryo and that grows, then sloughs off monthly, over the course of the menstrual cycle.

3. That the operation turned out to be "unnecessary" doesn't mean it was "negligent." The practice of medicine is replete with judgment calls—balances between risks that are impossible to estimate precisely—and decisions that turn out "wrong" from an after-the-fact perspective are inevitable.

4. D. Keith Edmonds, ed., *Dewhurst's Textbook of Obstetrics and Gynaecology,* 7th ed. (Malden, MA: Blackwell Publishing, 2007), 94.

5. Ibid., 431.

6. They've done so since the 1920s, when a gynecologist named John Sampson offered it up, without actually showing that women menstruate into their insides. Sampson, J.A. "Peritoneal endometriosis due to the menstrual dissemination of endometrial tissue into the peritoneal cavity," *American Journal of Obstetrics and Gynecology* 14 (1927): 422–469.

7. David B. Redwine, "Diaphragmatic Endometriosis: Diagnosis, Surgical Management and Long-Term Results of Treatment" *Fertility and Sterility* 77, issue 2 (February 2002): 288–296; Richard Brouwer and Rodney J. Woods, "Rectal Endometriosis: Results of Radical Excision and Review of Published Work," *ANZ Journal of Surgery* 77, issue 7 (July 2007): 562–571. Of those with recurring pain, Redwine and his colleagues claim, a large majority are "cured"—that is, they stay symptom-free—by follow-on surgery to remove all visible endometrial growths.

8. Members of the Sutter Independent Physicians network, with which Carrie's HMO, HealthNet, contracts for care, are scored on a point system, based on measures of clinical quality (e.g., percentages of their patients who receive recommended pap smears, mammograms, etc.) and frugality. They receive twice-a-year incentive payments based on these scores. Interview with Jennifer Hopper, Carrie's primary care physician.

9. Interview with Dr. Jennifer Hopper, September 2, 2008.

10. J. E. Wennberg and A. Gittlesohn, "Small Area Variations in Healthcare Delivery," *Science* 182 (1973): 1102–1108.

11. JoAnn E. Manson, MD, et al., "Estrogen plus Progestin and the Risk of Coronary Heart Disease," *New England Journal of Medicine* 349, no. 6 (August 2003): 523–534.

12. William E. Boden, MD, et al., "Optimal Medical Therapy with or without PCI for Stable Coronary Disease," *New England Journal of Medicine* 356, no. 15 (April 2007): 1503–1516. Stents prevent heart attacks (and save lives), it turned out, when they are

placed in the coronary arteries of patients with unstable angina, an indicator of active clot formation. But stenting stable blockages—stretches of atherosclerotic plaque where clots aren't quickly forming—yields no such benefit; to the contrary, it adds to cardiac risk.

13. The main exception is care that's specifically excluded by contract: common exclusions include *in vitro* fertilization, liver transplants, and limits on mental hospitalization.

14. *Pegram v. Herdrich,* 530 U.S. 211 (2000).

15. *Herdrich v. Pegram,* 154 F. 3d 362 (1998), quoting "For Our Patients, Not for Profits: A Call to Action," *Journal of the American Medical Association* 278 (1997): 1733–1738.

16. 530 U.S. at 220–221.

17. Herdrich also sued Pegram for medical malpractice (for not obtaining an ultrasound more quickly); Herdrich and Pegram settled the malpractice action for $30,000.

18. I tried to persuade the Justices to do so, by co-authoring an amicus brief in the case, signed by 35 health law and policy scholars, calling upon the Court to take account of physicians' Hippocratic duty to keep faith with patients.

19. 530 U.S. at 221.

20. Sarah Palin famously transmuted proposed Medicare coverage for end-of-life counseling into a "death panel" empowered to decide who shall live based on "level of productivity in society." Marc Ambinder, "Zeke Emanuel, The Death Panels, and Illogic in Politics," *The Atlantic,* August 11, 2009, available at http://www.theatlantic.com/politics/archive/2009/08/zeke-emanuel-the-death-panels-and-illogic-in-politics/23088/. The origin of the "rationing boards" canard is obscure, but Rush Limbaugh gave it a boost by so characterizing a federal panel tasked with overseeing research into the comparative effectiveness of clinical tests and treatments.

21. The Hippocratic Oath, Congresswoman and "Tea Party" icon Michele Bachmann (R-MN) said in a much-cited speech on the floor of the House of Representatives, is "an imperative to do everything for the patient regardless of the cost or effects on others." The proposition that doctors should count costs, she asserted, "is a horrific notion to our nation's doctors [and] to each American." 155.114 Cong. Rec. H8851-H8852 (July 27, 2009)(Statement of Rep. Bachmann) available at: http://frwebgate.access.gpo.gov/cgi-bin/getpage.cgi?dbname=2009_record&page=H8811&position=all.

22. The 30 percent figure comes from work by a team of Dartmouth University researchers renown in health policy circles for their study of wide variations in clinical practice and of the cost-effectiveness of tests and treatments. Megan McAndrew, MBA, MS, and Kristen K. Bronner, MA, eds., *The Care of Patients with Severe Chronic Illness: An Online Report of the Medicare Program by the Dartmouth Atlas Project* (2006). http://www.dartmouthatlas.org/downloads/atlases/2006_Chronic_Care_Atlas.pdf

23. The 2010 health reform law creates such a program, to be overseen by a panel of clinical researchers and health care industry representatives and jointly funded by government and industry. The Patient Protection and Affordable Care Act of 2010, H.R. 3590, Part III Subtitle D, "Patient-Centered Outcomes Research" § 6301, 6302.

24. M. Gregg Bloche, "The Invention of Health Law," *California Law Review* 91 (March 2003): 247–322.

25. HealthNet's contract permitted it to count cost only when "an alternative [cheaper] service or sequence of services [is] at least as likely to produce equivalent therapeutic or diagnostic results. . . ." The contract also required that care be in accord with "standards [of medical practice] that are based on credible scientific evidence published in peer-reviewed medical literature generally recognized by the relevant medical community."

26. In California and more than 40 other states, laws enacted since the mid-1990s empower patients to obtain independent medical review of coverage denials. See *Rush-Prudential HMO, Inc. v. Moran,* 536 U.S. 355 (2002). Patients, their doctors, and insurers submit

clinical records and other supporting evidence to panels of physicians with no financial or other stake in the outcome. These panels then make coverage determinations that are, for practical purposes, binding on patients, doctors, and insurers.

27. These included the absence of controls (that is, patients assigned to conventional surgical and drug therapies) and the fact that patients weren't randomly selected for the more aggressive approach.

28. Beta HCG levels are reported in milli-international units per milliliter (mIU/ml).

29. Kip Viscusi, "The Value of Risks to Life and Health," *Journal of Economic Literature* 31, no. 4 (December 1993): 1912–1946; W. Kip Viscusi, "Mortality Effects of Regulatory Costs and Policy Evaluation Criteria," *The RAND Journal of Economics* 25, no. 1 (Spring 1994): 94–109.

30. Restatement 2nd of Torts: Negligence § 328 (1965).

31. See American College of Emergency Physicians, "Clinical Policy for the Initial Approach to Adolescents and Adults Presenting to the Emergency Department With a Chief Complaint of Headache," *Annals of Emergency Medicine* 27, no. 6 (June 1996): 821–844.

32. David J. Brenner & Eric J. Hall, "Computerized Tomography—An Increasing Source of Radiation Exposure," *New England Journal of Medicine* 357 (2007): 2277–2284.

33. Department of Emergency Medicine, *Student Manual,* p. 31, Medical College of Georgia (2004).

34. Ibid.

35. Robert A. Smith, "The Evolving Role of MRI in the Detection & Evaluation of Breast Cancer," *New England Journal of Medicine* 356 (2007): 1362.

36. Debbie Saslow et al., *American Cancer Society Guidelines for Breast Screening with MRI as an Adjunct to Mammography, CA: A Cancer Journal for Clinicians* 57 (2007): 75–89.

37. Clinical practice guidance from highly-regarded bodies like the American Cancer Society carries much weight in court (in suits over denial of coverage) and with independent medical review panels (created by law in more than 40 states to hear appeals when insurers decline coverage). Guidelines from such bodies also put market pressure on health plans by creating reputational costs for plans that refuse to pay for recommended tests and treatments.

38. The "Guidelines" do, though, include an escape valve. They don't explicitly advise *against* MRI screening for women who aren't at high-risk; instead, they recommend it for women who *are.* This leaves room for doctors to order the test for lower-risk women who are financially well-off and willing and able to pay for it out-of-pocket. The unspoken consequence is a two-tiered system of early cancer detection, tied to personal wealth.

39. The case was presented by an HMO staff member for discussion at the retreat. "Sarah Eisenberg" is a pseudonym. I was given permission to write about this episode (and to interview some of the principals) on condition that I keep the identities of the patient, her caregivers and family members, and the HMO anonymous.

40. "Lisa" is a pseudonym."

41. Her doctors hypothesized about so-called "hibernating myocardium"—cardiac muscle that doesn't die but that temporarily stops working after a heart attack (for hours or days) while it recovers from stress.

42. Thaddeus Mason Pope, "Medical Futility Statutes: No Safe Harbor to Unilaterally Refuse Life Sustaining Treatment," *Tennessee Law Review* 75 (Fall 2007): 1–82.

43. Ibid. See also M. Wreen, "Medical Futility and Physician Discretion," *Journal of Medical Ethics* 30, no. 3 (June 2004): 275–278; Thomas Wm. Mayo, "Living and Dying in a Post-Schiavo World," *Journal of Health Law* 38, no. 4 (2005): 587–608; Ashley Bassel,

"Order at the End of Life: Establishing a Clear and Fair Mechanism for the Resolution of Futility Disputes," *Vanderbilt Law Review* 63 (March 2010): 491–540.

44. Vernon's Texas Statutes and Codes Annotated, Health & Safety Code § 166.046.

45. Schneiderman defines success as restoration of consciousness, elimination of total dependence on ICU life support, or other improvement in life circumstances.

46. Lawrence J. Schneiderman, Nancy S. Jecker, and Albert R. Jonsen, "Medical Futility: Its Meaning and Ethical Implications," in *Bioethics: An Introduction to the History, Methods, and Practice,* 2d ed., Nancy S. Jecker, Albert R. Jonsen, and Robert A. Pearlman, eds. (Sudbury, MA: Jones and Bartlett Publishers, 2007): 408–416.

47. Mark Hall "Law, Medicine, & Trust," *Stanford Law Review* 55 (2002): 463.

48. Mark D. Hauser. Moral Minds: How Nature Designed our Universal Sense of Right and Wrong (New York: Ecco, 2006).

Chapter Three   Stakeholders, Wonks, and the Setting of Limits

1. See McAndrew, *supra* chapter 2 n. 22.

2. Office of Technology Assessment *Assessing the Efficacy and Safety of Medical Technologies,* September 1978.

3. Shannon Brownlee, *Overtreated: Why Too Much Medicine is Making us Sicker and Poorer* (New York: Bloomsbury, 2007): 293.

4. Once known as the Agency for Health Care Policy & Research (AHCPR) (when it had the power to issue evidence-based clinical practice guidelines), it was reconstituted in 1999 in downsized form as the Agency for Healthcare Research & Quality (AHRQ) and barred from issuing clinical guidelines that could become a basis for withholding insurance coverage. http://www.ahrq.gov/about/ahrqfact.htm

5. My account, in this paragraph, of the battle over Medicare coverage for CT angiography relies upon Julia Appleby's superb account. Julia Appleby, "The Case of CT Angiography: How Americans View and Embrace New Technology," *Health Affairs* 27 (2008): 1515.

6. The agency, the Centers for Medicare & Medicaid Services (CMS) said it would cover the scans only for patients with symptoms of insufficient blood flow to the heart (typically chest pain or discomfort, known as angina, associated with physical exertion or emotional stress). CMS thereby excluded a broad range of patients who'd been receiving the scans, including symptomless patients with cardiac risk factors (e.g., elevated low-density lipoproteins) and even worried people seeking reassurance, absent any risk factors.

7. Alex Berenson and Reed Abelson, "The Evidence Gap: Weighing the Costs of a CT Scan's Look Inside the Heart," *The New York Times* June 29. 2008.

8. The Food and Drug Administration (FDA) requires drug and device makers to show that their products are "safe" and "effective"; this standard permits the companies to put pricey new products on the market without a showing that they represent improvement over existing, cheaper therapies. Studies designed by these firms (or researchers acting on their behalf) with this regulatory requirement in mind rarely look at how new products stack up to existing options. The drug and device makers have long opposed legislation requiring them to show that new, patent-protected products have superior efficacy in order to win FDA approval. New surgical and other procedures can enter medical practice without a showing that they're "safe" and "effective"—their adoption is constrained only by physicians' willingness to prescribe them and insurers' willingness to pay.

9. Hormone replacement, once thought to reduce post-menopausal women's risk of fatal cardiovascular events (heart attacks and strokes), turned out to increase it. See Manson, *supra* chapter 2 n. 11. Drug-coated screens (stents) in coronary arteries likewise turned

out to raise the risk of fatal vascular events—except when placed in arteries on an emergency basis, to push back against actively-forming clots. See Boden, *supra* chapter 2 n. 12.

10. Jeffrey A. Lieberman, M.D. et al., "Effectiveness of Antipsychotic Drugs in Patients with Chronic Schizophrenia," *New England Journal of Medicine* 353, no. 12 (September 2005): 1209–1223.

11. For example, the Patient Protection and Affordable Care Act provides that "Nothing in section 1181 [which addresses comparative clinical effectiveness research] shall be construed as . . . authorizing the Secretary to deny coverage of items or services under such title solely on the basis of comparative clinical effectiveness research." Patient Protection and Affordable Care Act, Pub. L. No. 111–148, §1182(b)(2), 937 Stat. 622 (2010).

12. Like drugs themselves, many clinical trials have been given catchy names (actually acronyms) in recent years by researchers looking for "branding" as a way to attract attention amidst a cacophony of medical information. "Allhat" stands for "Antihypertensive and Lipid-Lowering Treatment to Prevent Heart Attack Trial."—and, of course, for a horseriding Western wanna-be who (like a brand-name drug that proves less effective than a generic) doesn't quite measure up.

13. ALLHAT Collaborative Research Group, "Major Outcomes in High-Risk Hypertensive Patients Randomized to Angiotensin-Converting Enzyme Inhibitor or Calcium Channel Blocker vs. Diuretic," *Journal of the American Medical Association* 288, no. 23 (December 2002): 2981–2997. The study found that the fifty-year-old thiazide diuretic did as well as or better than its newer, patented rivals at controlling blood pressure and reducing the occurrence of cardiovascular diseases.

14. Andrew Pollack, "The Evidence Gap: The Minimal Impact of a Big Hypertension Study," *New York Times,* November 28, 2008.

15. Ibid. The e-mail was obtained by lawyers for patients who sued the company, then made available to the journalist Andrew Pollack.

16. Ibid.

17. Similarly, "Cardura" sales trailed off after 2000, when Pfizer reduced its promotional commitment after this drug lost patent protection.

18. This drug, also marketed by Merck, raised the risk of heart failure by nearly 20 percent (compared to the diuretic) and made strokes 15 percent more likely.

19. Phillip Anderson, "Complexity Theory and Organization Science," *Organization Science* 10, no. 3, Special Issue: Application of Complexity Theory (May/June 1999): 216–232.

20. Most obviously, the insurance industry (perhaps the most potent lobby in Washington) opposes its own demise; others allied against the "single payer" approach include medical societies, hospitals, and drug and device makers, all of which fear, with good reason, that a "single payer" would wield its purchasing power to push down prices.

21. During the course of the 2009–10 debate over health care reform, "bending the curve" became the fashionable phrase for long-term cost containment. It first appeared as the title to a health policy think tank's 2007 report on health spending. Cathy Schoen, Stuart Guterman, Anthony Shih, Jennifer Lau, Sophie Kasimow, Anne Gauthier, and Karen Davis, *Bending the Curve: Options for Achieving Savings and Improving Value in Health Spending* (New York: Commonwealth Fund, 2007). That the report didn't live up to its title (it offered sensible proposals for getting more value from our health care spending but shied away from suggesting strategies for restraining the pricey technological advances that power the cost curve's long-term rise), is, itself, testimony to the difficulty of speaking in polite company about the medical limit-setting challenge the U.S. faces.

22. Francis T. McAndrew, "New Evolutionary Perspectives on Altruism: Multilevel-Selection and Costly-Signaling Theories," *Current Directions in Psychological Science* 11, no. 2 (April 2002): 79–82.
23. Lewis Thomas, "On the Science and Technology of Medicine," *Daedalus—Doing Better and Feeling Worse: Health in the United States* 106, no. 1 (Winter 1977): 35–46.
24. Invasive cardiologists, for example, averaged $460,000 in income in 2007, compared to $365,000 for non-invasive cardiologists. Martin, Fletcher Annual Benefits and Compensation Report (2007), http://www.martinfletcher.com/PressRoom/MF_CompSurvey_Phys_07.pdf. Similar pay gaps, tied to the invasiveness and technological intensity of tests and treatments, pervade medicine.
25. Medical costs as a percentage of GDP will rise for the foreseeable future, pushed upwards by biomedical breakthroughs, longer life-spans, and, of course, insurance that desensitizes patients to the costs of innovation.
26. Attempts to eliminate doctors' discretion by promulgating rules in exhaustive detail are bound to backfire, by confusing doctors (through opacity and contradiction) to the point that they end up exercising *broader,* less confined discretion and by compelling absurd, unanticipated clinical consequences.
27. *Rule 3.1* of the American Bar Association's *Model Rules of Professional Conduct* (2004) states that: "A lawyer shall not bring or defend a proceeding, or assert or controvert an issue therein, unless there is a basis in law and fact for doing so that is not frivolous, which includes a good faith argument for an extension, modification or reversal of existing law."
28. Doctors will still exercise plenty of discretionary judgment within these principles' interstices. Medicine's myriad uncertainties ensure a wide berth for professional judgment when doctors apply these principles to actual cases; moreover, such principles can't come close to anticipating all clinical circumstances in advance.
29. In economics language, the premise here is that medical care is a "merit good"—a product or service for which ability and willingness to pay aren't the proper distributive guideposts. Among the justifications often given for treating health care this way is that valuing a person's health based on her wealth is an affront to human dignity (or to our ideals about equity), that health is essential to human functioning (including pursuit of economic opportunity), Normal Daniels, *Just Health Care: Studies in Philosophy and Health Policy* (New York: Cambridge University Press, 1985), and that access to adequate medical care is a marker of membership in a polity (at least in the industrialized world). Michael Walzer, *Spheres of Justice: A Defense of Pluralism and Equality* (New York: Basic Books, Inc., 1983).
30. The "Federal Health Board" proposed by Secretary of Health and Human Services Thomas Daschle, is one prototype. See Tom Daschle, Scott S. Greenberger, and Jeanne M. Lambrew, *Critical: What we can do about the Health Care Crisis* (New York: Thomas Dunne Books, 2008). Daschle's board would develop binding coverage principles and rules, shielded from administrative and legal challenge. The UK's National Institute for Clinical Effectiveness (NICE) and Germany's Institute for Quality and Efficiency in Health Care (IQWiG) represent an alternative model: NICE and IQWiG give stakeholders (including medical specialists, hospitals, drug and device makers, and patient advocacy organizations) some voice, in the form of opportunities to make public submissions and to appeal initial coverage decisions. Neither NICE nor IQWiG aim to base their coverage protocols on explicit cost-benefit trade-off principles. Instead, both take current therapies as givens and ask whether innovations offer substantial improvement in outcomes in return for their higher costs.
31. Clark C. Havighurst, *Health Care Choices: Private Contracts as Instruments of Health Reform* (Washington, D.C.: American Enterprise Institute, 1995).

Chapter Four   Politics, Morals, and Medical Need I: PTSD

1. The Pentagon's practice was and is to fly soldiers for free only to international arrival points in the US; soldiers and their families were then responsible for the costs of getting to their homes.

2. Zahara Solomon and Mario Mikulincer, "Trajectories of PSTD: A 20 Year Longitudinal Study," *American Journal of Psychiatry* 163, issue 4 (2006): 659–666; Edgar Jones, Robert Hodgins_Vermaas, Helen McCartney, Brian Everitt, Charlotte Beech, Denise Poynter, Ian Palmer, Kenneth Hyams, Simon Wessely, "Post_combat syndromes from the Boer war to the Gulf war: a cluster analysis of their nature and attribution," *British Medical Journal* 324 (2002): 1–7.

3. American Psychiatric Association: *Diagnostic and Statistical Manual*, Fourth Edition, Text Revision (Washington, D.C.: American Psychiatric Association, 2000), 463–467.

4. The *TR* stands for "Text Revision": minor changes were made to the *DSM–4* in 2000.

5. The APA's agreement on diagnostic categories and criteria was published in 1980 as the *Diagnostic and Statistical Manual of Mental Disorders, 3rd Edition (DSM–3)*. Revisions were published in 1987 (the *DSM–3-R, or Diagnostic and Statistical Manual of Mental Disorders, 3rd Edition, Revised*), 1994 (the *DSM–4*), and 2000 (the *DSM–4-TR*). A fifth edition is expected out in 2013.

6. Although combat trauma inspired the development of PTSD as a diagnostic category, the APA manual's drafters intended PTSD to be more broad-reaching: torture, war atrocities, rape, and other violent crimes were among the traumatic experiences said to be capable of inducing the syndrome. In the language of the manual, PTSD can ensue if "the person experienced, witnessed, or was confronted with an event or events that involved actual or threatened death or serious injury, or a threat to the physical integrity of self or others" and "the person's response involved intense fear, helplessness, or horror." American Psychiatric Association: *Diagnostic and Statistical Manual*, Fourth Edition, Text Revision (Washington, D.C.: American Psychiatric Association, 2000), 463, 467.

7. Ben Shepherd, *A War of Nerves, Soldiers and Psychiatrists in the Twentieth Century* (Cambridge, MA: Harvard University Press 2001); Sally Satel, MD and B. Christopher Frueh, PhD, "Sociopolitical Aspects of Psychiatry" in *Kaplan and Sadock's Comprehensive Textbook of Psychiatry: Ninth Edition Vol. 1,* Benjamin James Sadock, MD, Virginia Alcott Sadock, MD, and Pedro Ruiz, MD, eds. (Philadelphia: Lippincott Williams & Wilkins, 2009), 728–734.

8. Sally Satel, "Stressed Out Vets: Believing the Worst About Post-Traumatic Stress Disorder," *The Weekly Standard* 11, no. 46 (August 11, 2006).

9. Shankar Vedantam, "A Political Debate on Stress Disorder," *Washington Post*, December 27, 2005.

10. Charles S. Milliken et al., "Longitudinal Assessment of Mental Health Problems among Active and Reserve Component Soldiers Returning from the Iraq War," *Journal of the American Medical Association* 298, no.18 (2007): 2141–2148.

11. Report of the Mental Health Advisory Team V, Office of the Surgeon Multi-National Force: Iraq, Office of the Command Surgeon, and Office of the Surgeon General U.S. Army Medical Command (February 14, 2008), http://www.armymedicine.army.mil/reports/mhat/mhat_v/MHAT_V_OIFandOEF-Redacted.pdf.

12. Joseph E. Stiglitz and Linda J. Bilmes, *The Economic Cost of the Iraq War*, Milken Institute, 4th Quarter (2006); Congressional Joint Economic Committee, *War at any Price: The Total Economic Costs of the War Beyond the Federal Budget* (2007).

13. Atul Gawande, MD, MPH, "Casualties of War—Military Care for the Wounded from Iraq and Afghanistan," *The New England Journal of Medicine* 351, no. 24 (2004): 2471–2475.

14. Dept. of Veterans Affairs, Office of Public Affairs, *America's Wars,* September 30, 2006. http://www1.va.gov/opa/publications/factsheets/fs_americas_wars.pdf.

15. Linda Bilmes, "Soldiers Returning Home from Iraq and Afghanistan: The Long-Term Costs of Providing Veterans Medical Car and Disability Benefits," (Working Paper 07–001, Harvard University, John F. Kennedy School of Government, Faculty Research, 2007).

16. J. Alexander Bodkin, Harrison G. Pope· Michael J. Detke and James 1. Hudson, "Is PSTD Caused by Traumatic Stress," *Journal of Anxiety Disorders* 21, issue 2 (2007): 176–182.

17. Karen H. Seal, "Trends and Risk Factors for Mental Health Diagnosis among Iraq and Afghanistan Veterans using Department of Veteran Affairs Health Care, 2002–2008," *American Journal of Public Health* 99, no. 9 (2009): 1651–1658.

18. Michael De Yoana and Mark Benjamin, "Coming Home, the Army's Fatal Neglect," *Salon,* April 8, 2009.

19. Kelly Kennedy, "Fort Carson Faces more Probes into PSTD Cases," *Army Times,* May 4, 2010, http://www.armytimes.com/news/2007/05/military_carson_070503w/; Daniel Zwerdling, Soldiers Say Army Ignores, Punishes Mental Anguish, *National Public Radio,* December 4, 2004, http://www.npr.org/templates/story/story.php?storyId=6576505.

20. Joshua Kors, "How Specialist Town Lost His Benefits," *The Nation,* April 9, 2007.

21. Kelly Kennedy, "VA Officials Grilled on PTSD E-Mail," *Army Times,* June 10, 2008, http://www.armytimes.com/benefits/health/military_wounds_061008w/.

22. U.S. Army regulations permit involuntary discharge based on diagnosis of a "personality disorder" by a psychiatrist or psychologist, recommendation (by the psychiatrist or psychologist) that the soldier be discharged, and agreement by the soldier's commanding officer. AR 635–200, Chapter 5–13 (Personality Disorder).

23. Had Dr. Gray given Cruz a PTSD diagnosis, a narrative summary of his case *might* then have been sent to an Army "Medical Evaluation Board" for a determination of fitness for duty. A determination of unfitness would have led to a "medical discharge" (making him immediately eligible for VA medical care) and triggered an assessment of level of disability by a "Physical Evaluation Board." A disability rating of 30 percent or more would have qualified Cruz for a monthly Army disability payment for life (ratings below 30 percent result in denial of disability benefits). This process takes six months to a year, according to military medical sources with whom I've spoken. A medical discharge isn't finalized until the Physical Evaluation Board issues its rating; until this happens, the service member remains in a sort of administrative limbo, paid by the military but unable to continue his career. By contrast, a Chapter 5–13 discharge is typically complete within a few to several months of the psychiatrist's or psychologist's recommendation. This makes the "medical discharge" route more costly for the military than the Chapter 5–13 path. But Chapter 5–13 not only ensures denial of medical and disability benefits; it results in a so-called "general discharge," potentially damaging to a veteran's pursuit of opportunities in civilian life.

24. We're hypocritical about this, of course: markets for pornography and prostitution thrive (on both sides of the law), and sexual contact between film stars has become a mainstay of middle-American movie-going. But porn and prostitution remain in disrepute, and sex on the big screen is shielded from judgment by a measure of artistic conceit.

25. Dr. Ben Phillips, chief of behavior health at Ft Hood (and Dr. Grey's supervisor) declined to discuss the diagnosis of PTSD and personality disorder with me when I phoned him. Other army behavioral health leaders have likewise refused to speak for the record about their guidance to clinicians concerning PTSD and personality disorder diagnosis.

26. Letter to The Hon. Dr. Robert Gates, Secretary of Defense from Senators Kit Bond, Barbara Boxer, Joseph Lieberman and Barack Obama June 21, 2007, http://grassley. senate.gov/about/upload/Secretary-Gates-letter.pdf. The letter was also signed by: Max Baucus (D-MT), Evan Bayh (D-IN), Joseph Biden (D-DE), Maria Cantwell (D-WA), Benjamin Cardin (D-MD), Hillary Clinton (D-NY), Susan Collins (R-ME), Christopher Dodd (D-CT), Elizabeth Dole (R-NC), Russell Feingold (D-WI), Charles Grassley (R-IA), Judd Gregg (R-NH), Tom Harkin (D-IA), Edward Kennedy (D-MA), John Kerry (D-MA), Herb Kohl (D-WI), Frank Lautenberg (D-NJ), Patrick Leahy (D-VT), Claire McCaskill (D-MO), Barbara Mikulski (D-MD), Patty Murray (D-WA), Bernard Sanders (I-VT), Olympia Snowe (R-ME), John Sununu (R-NH), Jon Tester (D-MT), Ron Wyden (D-OR).

27. Interview with Senator Kit Bond (R-MO), Congressman Bob Filner (D-CA), and musician Dave Matthews by Bob Woodruff, ABC Nightline Segment, July 12, 2007).

28. Audio available at: http://joshuakors.com/davematthews042207.mp3

29. Office of the Undersecretary of Defense for Personnel and Readiness, *Report to Congress on Administrative Separations Based on Personality Disorder: Fiscal Years 2002 thru 2007* 10 (2008): 10.

30. Abraham Lincoln, Inaugural Address March 4, 1865, *The Abraham Lincoln Papers at the Library of Congress, Section 3. General Correspondence (1837–1897),* http://memory.loc.gov/cgi-bin/ampage?collId=mal&fileName=mal3/436/4361300/malpage. db&recNum=0.

Chapter Five   Politics, Morals, and Medical Need II: Mobilizing Shared Resources

1. American Psychiatric Association: *Diagnostic and Statistical Manual,* Fourth Edition, Text Revision (Washington, D.C.: American Psychiatric Association, 2000), p. 683.

2. Ibid.

3. Ibid., 717.

4. Doris Kearns Goodwin, *Team of Rivals: The Political Genius of Abraham Lincoln* (New York: Simon & Schuster, 2005), pp. 5–59.

5. "Idiopathic" is the Latin-derived term doctors use to refer to a condition without a known cause.

6. Joyce M. Lee, Matthew M. Davis, et al., "Estimated Cost-effectiveness of Growth Hormone Therapy for Idiopathic Short Stature," *Archives of Pediatric & Adolescent Medicine* 160, no. 3.(2006): 263–269.

7. G. A. Bray, "Obesity Is a Chronic, Relapsing Neurochemical Disease," *International Journal of Obesity* 28, no. 1 (2004): 34–38.

8. Oft-cited causes of epidemic obesity include declining food prices and rising incomes, sedentary employment and exurban sprawl, TV and video games, on-line social networking, larger portion sizes, shorter food preparation times, tempting fast-food ads, and even (more controversially) movement of women into the workplace. Substantial evidence supports some of these purported causes; evidence for others is dubious. Susan Okie, *Winning the War against Childhood Obesity* (Washington D.C.: Joseph Henry Press, 2005); Eric A. Finklestein & Laurie Zuckerman, *The Fattening of America: How the Economy Makes Us Fat, If It Matters, and What to Do About It* (Hoboken, NJ: John Wiley & Sons, Inc. 2008); David Crawford, Robert W. Jeffrey, Kylie Ball, and Johannes Brug, eds., *Obesity Epidemiology: From Aetiology to Public Health, Second Edition* (Oxford: Oxford University Press, 2010).

9. The difficulty of measuring body fat as a percentage of people's total weight, case by case, has led medicine to embrace the Body Mass Index (BMI) as a surrogate measure of

body fat. BMI = weight (in kilograms)/height (in meters)^2. By convention, people with BMIs greater than 25 are overweight; those with BMIs greater than 30 are obese.

10. Richard Epstein, "What (Not) to do About Obesity: A Moderate Aristotelian Answer," *Georgetown Law Journal* 93, no. 4 (2005): 1361.

11. Both supporters and critics of the obesity-as-disease proposition have claimed that science takes their side. Backers point to its biological causes (breakdowns in feedback loops that regulate appetite) and consequences (increased risk for life-shortening and disabling illnesses), agreed-upon clinical signs (BMI, waist circumference, and, in severe cases, metabolic derangements), and treatments (diet and exercise, medications, and even surgery to remove parts of the digestive tract). Critics say that its neurochemical determinants are ill-understood, that there's no natural distinction between those who are and aren't afflicted (we all store food energy in fat cells; BMI and waist circumference thresholds are arbitrary criteria), and it exhibits no symptoms (it may cause illnesses with symptoms but it's not, in itself, such an illness). But medicine treats other syndromes with poorly-understood determinants as diseases (e.g., cancers, depression). And a variety of conditions recognized as illnesses lack natural distinctions between those who are and aren't affected—consider, for example, hypertension (we all have blood pressures, just as we all have fat cells, and the dividing line between what's normal and elevated is drawn by the medical profession). Likewise, hypertension and some other syndromes accepted as illnesses lack symptoms; they're clinically significant only because they contribute to the later development of disabling or life-threatening health problems.

12. The agency, the Center for Medicare & Medicaid Services (CMS), didn't say it would immediately cover treatment for obesity; rather, CMS said it would henceforth consider covering particular therapies if patients and providers could present scientific proof of their efficacy.

13. Rick Berman, executive director of the Center for Consumer Freedom, quoted in Rob Stein and Ceci Connolly, "Medicare Changes Policy on Obesity," *Washington Post,* July 16, 2004, http://www.washingtonpost.com/wp-dyn/articles/A52835–2004Jul15.html.

14. American Obesity Association, *Medicare & Obesity: Frequently Asked Questions,* http://obesity1.tempdomainname.com/treatment/medicarefaq.shtml.

15. Dr. Joel Fuhrman, MD, Disease Proof (blog), http://www.diseaseproof.com/archives/2009/01/articles/cholesterol/.

16. Christiane Northrup, MD, "Buyer Beware: Statins to Lower Cholesterol Are Not a Panacea," http://www.huffingtonpost.com/christiane-northrup/buyer-beware-statins-are_b_246566.html.

17. Immunoglobulin E (Ig E) sets off asthma attacks by first binding to an antigen (a foreign material like pollen, dog dander, or dust mites), then binding to Ig E receptor molecules in the membranes of "mast cells." "Mast cells," in turn, release histamine and substances known as "cytokines." These, in turn, trigger inflammation and muscle spasms that narrow asthma sufferers' bronchi (tubes that carry air to and from the lungs), making it difficult for them to breath. "Omalizumab" blocks this process by attaching to Ig E molecules in a way that prevents Ig E from binding to receptors on "mast cells."

18. So-called "rescue" medications—inhaled or injected—will do this for several minutes, by inducing relaxation of muscles in patients' bronchi.

19. These drugs, known as corticosteroids, aren't the muscle-building steroids of sporting fame; they're a different family of steroids that depress immune responses.

20. National Asthma Education and Prevention Program, "Expert Panel Report 2: Guidelines for Diagnosis and Management of Asthma," *Journal of Allergy & Clinical Immunology* 110, no. 5 (2002): S141–S219.

21. R. J. Adams, A. Fuhlbrigge, et al., "Inadequate Use of Asthma Medication in the United States: Results of the Asthma in America National Population Survey," *Journal of Allergy & Clinical Immunology* 110, no. 1 (2002): 58–64.

22. Alarming numbers of Americans who have health insurance don't receive care that's in accord with recognized best practice. A RAND Corporation national survey, employing more than 400 evidence-based, best-practice measures, found a performance rate of only about 50 to 60 percent for most of these measures. Elizabeth A. McGlynn, Ph.D. et al, "The Quality of Health Care Delivered to Adults in the United States," *New England Journal of Medicine* 348 (June 26, 2003): 2635–2645.

23. Institute of Medicine, *Unequal Treatment: Confronting Racial and Ethnic Disparities in Health Care* (Washington, DC: National Academies Press, Washington, DC, 2003).

24. Gerd Gigerenzer et al., *Simple Heuristics that Make Us Smart* (New York: Oxford University Press, 2000).

25. The time-worn phrase, "art of medicine" captures this role.

26. Patricia A. King, *Dangers of Difference, in Tuskegee's Truths: Rethinking the Tuskegee Syphilis Study* (Chapel Hill, NC: University of North Carolina Press, 2000), pp. 424–430.

27. Juliet Lapidos, "The Aids Conspiracy Handbook: Jeremiah Wright's Paranoia, in Context," *Slate* (March 19, 2008), http://www.slate.com/id/2186860/.

28. Ibid.

29. Havighurst advised Ronald Reagan's 1980 campaign for the presidency.

30. Elliot S. Fischer, " Building a Medical Neighborhood for the Medical Home," *New England Journal of Medicine* 359, no. 1 (2008): 1202; Robert J. Reid et al., "The Group Health Medical Home at Year Two: Cost Savings, Higher Patient Satisfaction, and Less Burnout for Providers," *Health Affairs* 19, no. 5 (2010): 835; Sheryl M. Ness and William Young, "Dynamic Endocrine Testing: The Mayo Clinic Model," *Endocrinology & Metabolism Clinics of North America* 26, issue 4 (1997): 957–972.

31. The libertarian conservative scholar Richard Epstein points out that action on this front entails embedded cross-subsidies, and he's right. See Richard A. Epstein, "Disparities and Discrimination in Health Care Coverage: A Critique of the Institute of Medicine Study," *Perspectives in Biology and Medicine* 48 no. 1 Supplement (Winter 2005): 26. Efforts to reassure distrustful patients and their communities, forge connections with those most alienated from the health care system, and coordinate services for those least able to navigate through complex bureaucracies will require resources that are most likely to come from health insurance risk pools—and to thereby flow from the better-off to the least well-off among us.

Chapter Six   Setting Limits by Consent

1. "Mrs. Pearson" is a pseudonym.

2. Some physician-researchers claim there's no such compromise. So long as there's no scientific basis (before a comparative study is performed) for preferring the experimental or the conventional treatment, they argue, neither is better suited to a patient's needs.

3. Roy Porter, *The Greatest Benefit to Mankind: A Medical History of Humanity* 312–312 (1997).

4. English translation (from Spanish) of the Informed Consent Agreement for Antonio Benigno, November 26, 1900, Philip S. Hench Walter Reed Yellow Fever Collection, available at http://yellowfever.lib.virginia.edu/reed/data/7ed054b342c294297bdcb556 ddaddf0d.html.

5. The study saved hundreds of thousands of lives, maybe more, by pointing the way toward effective control of yellow fever through mosquito eradication campaigns in the American south, the Caribbean basin, Latin America, and elsewhere. It transformed

commerce and warfare by clearing the way for completion of the Panama Canal and ensuring that armies could maneuver in tropical environs without falling victim to this disease in enormous numbers.

6. Albert R. Jonsen, *The Birth of Bioethics* (New York: Oxford University Press, Inc., 1998): 129–133.

7. Hans-Martin Sass, "Reichsrundschreiben 1931: Pre-Nuremberg German Regulations Concerning New Therapy and Human Experimentation," *Journal of Medicine and Philosophy* (1983): 99–111.

8. Trials of War Criminals before the Nuremberg Military Tribunals under Control Council Law No. 10, Vol. 2, pp. 181–182. Washington, D.C.: U.S. Government Printing Office, 1949.

9. To be sure, by the 1940s, it had become common practice for American researchers to seek consent when they asked *healthy* people, not patients, to take part in experiments that put their lives or health at risk. *Advisory Committee on Human Radiation Experiments—Final Report* (1996): http://www.hss.energy.gov/HealthSafety/ohre/roadmap/achre/report.html.

10. Ibid.

11. Jay Katz, *Experimentation with Human Beings* (New York: Russel Sage Foundation, 1972).

12. See *Advisory Committee, supra* n. 9.

13. Katz, *supra* n. 11.

14. David J. Rothman, *Strangers at the Bedside: A History of How Law & Bioethics Transformed Medical Decision Making* (New York: Basic Books, Inc.,1991).

15. Michael B. Shimkin, "The Problem of Experimentation on Human Beings" *Science* Vol. 117 no. 3035 (February 1953): 205–215.

16. Peter D. Jacobson, *Strangers in the Night: Law and Medicine in the Managed Care Era* (New York: Oxford University Press, Inc., 2002); Charles E. Rosenberg, *The Care of Strangers: The Rise of America's Hospital System* (Baltimore: Johns Hopkins University Press, Inc., 1995); David J. Rothman, *Strangers at the Bedside: A History of How Law & Bioethics Transformed Medical Decision Making* (United States: Basic Books, 1991); Robert Burt, *Taking Care of Strangers: The Rule of Law in Doctor-Patient Relations* (New York: Free Press,1979).

17. National Institute of Health, *The Belmont Report: Ethical Principles and Guidelines for the Protection of Human Subjects of Research,* The National Commission for the Protection of Human Subjects of Biomedical and Behavioral Research (April 18, 1979): http://ohsr.od.nih.gov/guidelines/belmont.html.

18. The Tuskegee Syphilis Study, previously discussed, played a catalytic role in both the development of this framework and its incorporation into federal law. The Tuskegee revelations (and the federal inquiry that ensued) led Congress to create a National Commission for the Protection of Human Subjects of Biomedical and Behavioral Research. The Commission, composed of eminent clinicians, researchers, and scholars of medical ethics, announced three overarching moral principles—"respect for persons, beneficence, and justice." But, in practice, the first principle had paramount import: it translated into respect for autonomy and thus undergirded the requirement of informed consent. Or, so the Commission said, in an enormously influential document known as the *Belmont Report* (*supra* n. 17), which became the foundation for the federal regulatory framework that governs research medicine to this day.

19. Rothman, *supra* n. 14.

20. To be sure, insurance contracts from the 1970s and earlier contained coverage exclusions: most notably, insurers refused to cover "investigational" or "experimental"

therapies. But the question of "medical necessity" (the standard for coverage, absent a specific exclusion, in virtually all health insurance contracts) was the presumed province of the treating physician.

21. Commentators partial to this point drive it home with a standard metaphor: Ulysses binding himself to the mast to resist the allure of the Sirens.

22. *Shea v. Esensten,* 107 F.3d 625 (1997).

23. I say "presumably" because many Americans receive coverage from their employers and pay little out-of-pocket for it. Their employers pay most of the cost (a benefit that's tax-free for employees). Workers who decline this coverage can't opt to take their employers' share of its cost home as salary. They thus don't "feel" the full cost of coverage (and the care it buys), even at the sign-up stage.

24. Edmund Pellegrino, "Rationing Health Care : Conflicts within the Concept of Justice," in *The Ethics of Managed Care: Professional Integrity and Patient Rights,* eds. William B. Bondeson and James W. Jones, (Dordrecht: Kluwer Academic Publishers, 2002).

25. More precisely, fMRI measures variation in blood oxygen levels, which roughly track changes in blood flow and neuronal activity.

26. Colin F. Camerer and George Lowenstein, "Behavioral Economics: Past, Present, Future" in *Advances in Behavioral Economics,* Colin F. Camerer, George Lowenstein and Matthew Rabin, eds. (Princeton, N.J.: Princeton University Press, 2004): 3–53, 7.

27. Darcia Narvaez and Jenny L. Vaydich, "Moral Development and Behaviour under the Spotlight of the Neurobiological Sciences," *Journal of Moral Education* 37, issue 3 (2008): 289—312, 299.

28. Alan Wertheimer, *Coercion* (Princeton, NJ: Princeton University Press, 1987).

Chapter Seven   Doctors as Warriors I: America's Frisson with Torture

1. Telephone Interview with Scott Uithol (2010).

2. Department of Defense, *Taguba, Annex 46, Testimony of Colonel Thomas Pappas, Commander, 205th MI Brigade,* February 9, 2004, accessed October 28, 2010, www.aclu.org/torturefoia/released/a46.pdf.

3. Ibid.

4. M. Gregg Bloche and Jonathan H. Marks, "Triage at Abu Ghraib," *New York Times,* February 4, 2005.

5. Steven Miles, *An Oath Betrayed: America's Torture Doctors* (Berkeley and Los Angeles, CA: University of California Press, 2009), 54.

6. John D. Marks, *The Search for the Manchurian Candidate: The CIA and Mind Control* (New York: Norton, 1991), chap. 8.

7. Albert D. Biderman, Communist Attempts to Elicit False Confessions from Air Force Prisoners of War, *Bull. N.Y. Acad. Med.* 33:616–625 (1957).

8. Marks, a State Department bureaucrat turned journalist, has written perhaps the best account of the CIA's cold-war era efforts to put psychiatry and the behavioral sciences to use for national security purposes, including interrogation. See Marks, *supra* n. 6.

9. Ibid.

10. Ibid.

11. Numerous books and articles—some well-balanced and others more polemical—have recounted the CIA's Cold War sojourn into the use of science to reshape minds. These include Gordon Thomas, *Journey into Madness: The True Story of Secret CIA Mind Control and Medical Abuse* (New York: Bantam Books, 1990); Harvey Weinstein, *Psychiatry and the CIA: Victims of Mind Control* (Washington, DC: American Psychiatric Press, 1990); Ann Collins, *In the Sleep Room: The Story of the CIA Brainwashing Experiments in Canada* (Ontario, Canada: Key Porter Books, 1998).

12. CIA Inspector General's Office, *Report of Inspection of Mkultra/TSD,* July 26, 1963, 2.
13. Alfred McCoy, *A Question of Torture: CIA Interrogation from the Cold War to the War on Terror* (New York: Holt Paperbacks, 2006), 50.
14. Tim Weiner, "C.I.A. Taught, Then Dropped, Mental Torture in Latin America," *New York Times,* July 27, 1997; Gary Cohn et al., "Torture was Taught by CIA: Declassified Manual Details the Methods used in Honduras: Agency Denials Refuted," *Baltimore Sun,* January 27, 1997.
15. Lisa Haugaard, "Declassified Army and CIA Manuals An Analysis of their Content, Latin America Working Group," February 18, 1997, www.archivochile.com/Imperialismo/escu_ameri/USescamerica0010.pdf.
16. Central Intelligence Agency, "Kubark Counterintelligence Interrogation: July 1963," www.gwu.edu/~nsarchiv/NSAEBB/NSAEBB122/CIA%20Kubark%201-60.pdf; Central Intelligence Agency, "Human Resource Exploitation Training Manual (1983)," www.gwu.edu/~nsarchiv/NSAEBB/NSAEBB122/CIA%20Human%20Res%20Exploit%20A1-G11.pdf.
17. CIA, "Kubark Counterintelligence Interrogation," 99.
18. "Kubark" was the CIA's cryptonym, or code name, for itself.
19. Ibid.
20. Ibid.
21. Dana Priest, "U.S. Instructed Latins on Executions, Torture; Manuals uUsed 1982–91, Pentagon Reveals," *Washington Post,* September 21, 1996.
22. CIA Inspector General, "Special Review: [redacted] Counterterrorism Detention and Interrogation Activities, September 2001 to October 2003" (2004), www.aclu.org/torturefoia/released/052708/052708_Special_Review.pdf.
23. PREAL Operating Manual, Department of Justice—Office of Professional Responsibility, "Investigation into the Office of Legal Counsel's Memorandum Concerning Issues Relating to the Central Intelligence Agency's Use of 'Enhanced Interrogation Techniques' on Suspected Terrorists," July 29, 2009, 40. http://judiciary.house.gov/hearings/pdf/OPRFinalReport090729.pdf
24. "Talking paper" attached to 2007 JPRA memo from U.S. Air Force Colonel Brendan G. Clare to Navy and Marine Headquarters, quoted in Jeffrey Kaye, "Waterboarding Too Dangerous, Internal DoD Memo Reveals," Truthout.org, March 4, 2010. www.truthout.org/waterboarding-too-dangerous-internal-dod-memo-reveals57372
25. Ibid.
26. PREAL Operating Manual in Department of Justice, 40.
27. Martin Seligman and Steve Maier, "Failure to Escape Traumatic Shock," *Journal of Experimental Psychology* 74, no. 1 (1967).
28. Martin Seligman, *Learned Optimism: How to Change Your Mind and Your Life* (New York: Pocket Books, 1998); *The Optimistic Child: A Proven Program to Safeguard Children against Depression and Build Long-life Resilience* (New York: Harper Paperbacks 2007); *Authentic Happiness: Using the New Positive Psychology to Realize Your Potential for Lasting Fulfillment* (New York: Free Press, 2002).
29. Jesse Klein, "Cognitive Behavioral Therapy for Adolescents with Depression," *Evidence Based Mental Health* 11, no. 3 (2008), http://ebmh.bmj.com/content/11/3/76.full; Graeme Whitfield and Chris Williams, "The Evidence Base for Cognitive Behavioral Therapy in Depression Delivery in Busy Clinical Settings," *Advances in Psychiatric Treatment* 9, no. 1 (2009), http://apt.rcpsych.org/cgi/content/full/9/1/21.
30. Scott Shane, "Two U.S. Architects of Harsh Tactics in 9/11's Wake," *New York Times,* August 12, 2009.
31. Evelyne Shuster, "Fifty Years Later: The Significance of the Nuremberg Code," *New England Journal of Medicine* 337, no. 20 (1997): 1436.

32. Department of the Army, "Field Manual 34–52: Intelligence Interrogation," May 8, 1987, available at www.globalsecurity.org/intell/library/policy/army/fm/fm34–52/chapter3 .htm.

33. Katherine Eban, "The War on Terror: Rorschach and Awe," Vanity Fair.com, July 17, 2007, www.vanityfair.com/politics/features/2007/07/torture200707.

34. M. Gregg Bloche and Jonathan H. Marks, "Doing unto Others as They Did unto Us," *New York Times,* November 14, 2005.

35. My e-mail correspondence with Kirk Hubbard, from which I quote (and from which some of this discussion draws more generally) unfolded over two months during the spring of 2010).

36. Society for the Study of Peace, Conflict, and Violence, American Psychological Association Presidential Task Force on Psychological Ethics and National Security: Members' Biographical Statements (2005), www.clarku.edu/peacepsychology/tfpens.html.

37. Office of Inspector General, *Special Review: Counterterrorism Detention and Interrogation Activities,* (2004). www.aclu.org/torturefoia/released/052708/052708_Special _Review.pdf

38. U.S. Senate Committee on Armed Services, *Inquiry into the Treatment of Detainees in U.S. Custody,* November 20, 2008, 7.

39. Through his lawyer, Henry F. Schuelke, Mitchell declined to be interviewed for this book. (Schuelke cited ongoing criminal inquiries into the "enhanced" interrogation program.)

40. Senate Committee on Armed Services, *Inquiry,* 9.

41. Department of Justice, "Memorandum for Alberto R. Gonzales: Standards of Conduct for Interrogation under 18 U.S.C.§§ 2340–2340A," (2002), 13, www.gwu.edu/~nsarchiv/ NSAEBB/NSAEBB127/02.08.01.pdf.

42. See Shane, *supra* n. 30

43. Seligman didn't deny meeting with Mitchell and Jessen *before* his presentation to JPRA. And his insistence that he never "worked . . . on torture" means little, absent clear rejection of the Bush administration's capacious definition of this term.

44. More specifically, I asked Seligman: "I'd be very interested in your thinking re the role of psychologists (& psychology as a profession) in the development & promotion of this approach. Was the approach a plausible, if misguided, strategy for helping our country at a time of crisis, for which the psychologists involved should perhaps be criticized, but not condemned for misconduct, unethical behavior, etc. Or was development and promotion of this interrogation approach unethical—or otherwise professionally inappropriate? Your thoughts?"

45. Zubaydah was shot in the stomach, thigh, and one of his testicles during the raid that apprehended him. The CIA flew in a Johns Hopkins surgeon to treat him. See Scott Shane and Mark Mazzetti, "In Adopting Harsh Tactics, no Inquiry into Past Use," *New York Times* April 22, 2009.

46. Author's Spring 2010 E-Mail Correspondence with Kirk Hubbard.

47. U.S. Department of Justice, Office of the Inspector General, *A Review of the FBI's Involvement in and Observations of Detainee Interrogations in Guantanamo Bay, Afghanistan, and Iraq* (2008), 68–69. http://www.justice.gov/oig/special/s0910.pdf

48. James Mitchell, Psychological Assessment of Zain al-'Abedin al-Abideen Muhammad Hassan, a.k.a. Abu Zubaydah (2002). www.aclu.org/torturefoia/released/082409/ olcremand/2004olc4.pdf

49. Ibid.

50. The dairies, which spanned more than a decade, were taken in the raid that netted Zubaydah and immediately flown to CIA headquarters in McLean. CIA and FBI personnel who pored over a translated version found that he wrote in three different

"voices"—"Hani 1," "Hani 2," and "Hani 3"—aged twenty years apart, with different personalities. "This guy is insane, certifiable, split personality," one CIA analyst concluded. Ron Suskind, *The One Percent Doctrine* (New York: Simon and Schuster, 2007), 95–100. This was hardly enough to diagnose him with multiple personality disorder, but it was evidence that Zubaydah had a tendency to lapse into what psychiatrists call a "dissociative state"—a breakdown of the personality under stress, often accompanied by depression, severe anxiety, and reduced cognitive functioning. (Multiple personality is one kind of dissociative state.) SERE trainees who break down under the stresses of their mock captivity exhibit dissociative symptoms; indeed "dissociation" is the term psychiatrists associated with SERE typically use to describe this breakdown. Thus the dairies suggested that Zubaydah would be at unusually high risk for "severe mental pain and suffering" if exposed to SERE methods.

51. U.S. Department of Justice, Office of Professional Responsibility, *Report: Investigation Into the Office of Legal Counsel's Memoranda Concerning Issues Relating to the Central Intelligence Agency's Use of "Enhanced Interrogation Techniques" on Suspected Terrorists* (July 29, 2009). http://judiciary.house.gov/hearings/pdf/OPRFinalReport090729.pdf

52. David Margolis, Associate Deputy Attorney General, "Memorandum of Decision Regarding the Objections to the Findings of Professional Misconduct in the Office of Professional Responsibility's Report of Investigation Into the Office of Legal Counsel's Memoranda Concerning Issues Relating to the Central Intelligence Agency's Use of 'Enhanced Interrogation Techniques' on Suspected Terrorists" (January 5, 2010). http://judiciary.house.gov/hearings/pdf/DAGMargolisMemo100105.pdf

53. "Black sites" were secret CIA detention and interrogation facilities for post-9/11 detainees. A still-unrevealed number of "black sites" were scattered about Europe, Asia, and possibly elsewhere overseas.

54. Jay S. Bybee, "Memorandum for John Rizzo, Acting General Counsel of the Central Intelligence Agency: Interrogation of al Qaeda Operative" (August 1, 2002), 4, 11. http://www.globalsecurity.org/intell/library/policy/national/olc_08012002_bybee.pdf

55. Lawyers quibble about the precise definition of "specific intent." I've skipped the nuance here, but it's fair to say that treating "specific intent" as *purpose* is the mainstream approach.

56. Bybee, *supra* n. 54 at 16.

57. The CIA has acknowledged destroying all of its videos of enhanced interrogation, saying it did so out of fear that if the videos became public, widespread anger at the United States could undermine national security. The agency has so far declined (in Freedom of Information Act [FOIA] litigation, in which I am a plaintiff) to release interrogation logs and notes made by medical personnel.

58. Bybee, *supra* n. 54 at 3 – 4.

59. Brian Ross, "CIA—Abu Zubaydah, Interview with John Kiriakou," *CBS News: World Watch*, December 17, 2007, http://abcnews.go.com/images/Blotter/brianross_kiriakou_transcript1_blotter071210.pdf.

60. See Committee, *supra* n. 38 at 10–11.

61. Ibid. at 20–21.

62. See Inspector General, *supra* n. 22 at 31–32.

63. They were trained as torturers—that is, if one accepts prevailing international legal understandings of torture, which were, of course, at sharp variance with the Yoo-Bybee position.

64. "Walling" involved the pushing or throwing of detainees against a wall, said to be flexible to avoid injury.

65. More precisely, the text of one of the memos (defining "torture" and asserting presidential prerogative to authorize torture on behalf of national defense) became public in

2004. The existence of the other memo—the one approving use of SERE techniques on Zubaydah—was reported at the time, but its text was not made public until 2009, when the Obama administration agreed to its release in response to American Civil Liberties Union FOIA requests.

66. The most detailed of these memos, a 46 page exegesis on each technique's lawfulness (by Steven G. Bradbury, Bybee's successor as head of the OLC), couldn't have been clearer about CIA doctors' central role: "[T]he involvement of medical and psychological personnel in the adaptation and application of the established SERE techniques is particularly noteworthy for purposes of our analysis. Medical personnel have been involved in imposing limitations on—and requiring changes to—certain procedures, particularly the use of the waterboard. We have had extensive meetings with the medical personnel involved in monitoring the use of these techniques. It is clear that they have carefully worked to ensure that the techniques do not result in severe physical or mental pain or suffering to the detainees." See Steven G. Bradbury, "Memorandum for John Rizzo, Senior Deputy General Counsel, Central Intelligence Agency: Re: Application of 18 U.S.C. §§ 2340–2340A to the Combined Use of Certain Techniques in the Interrogation of High Value al Qaeda Detainees" (2005): 29 – 30, http://luxmedia.com. edgesuite.net/aclu/olc_05102005_bradbury46pg.pdf

67. Ibid. at 13–14.

68. Central Intelligence Agency, Office of Medical Services, "OMS Guidelines on Medical and Psychological Support to Detainee Rendition, Detention, and Interrogation" (2004), http://dspace.wrlc.org/doc/bitstream/2041/72435/02793_041200display.pdf

69. Ibid., 16.

70. Ibid., 17.

71. Bradbury, *supra* n. 66 at 40.

72. Robert E Roberts, Catherine Ramsay Roberts and Hao T. Duong, "Sleepness in Adolescence: Prospective Data on Sleep Deprivation, Health and Functioning," *Journal of Adolescence* 32, no. 5 (2009): 1045–1057; Michael A. Grander et al., "Problems Associated with Short Sleep: Bridging the Gap between Laboratory and Epidemiological Studies," *Sleep Medicine Reviews* 14, no. 4 (2009): 239; Varsha Taskar and Max Hirshkowitz, "Health Effects of Sleep Deprivation," *Clinical Pulmonary Medicine,* 10, no. 1 (2003): 47.

73. See Guidelines, *supra* n. 68 at 9–11.

74. United Nations, Principles of Medical Ethics, Resolution A/RES.37/194, December 18, 1982, www.un.org/documents/ga/res/37/a37r194.htm (emphasis added).

75. The OLC's interconnected set of May 2005 memos argued that the CIA's enhanced interrogation program didn't constitute torture under U.S. law and was neither torture nor "cruel, inhumane or degrading treatment" under international law (the Convention Against Torture and Other Cruel, Inhumane, or Degrading Treatment or Punishment). The OLC's detailed discussion of medical evidence and physician involvement as grounds for concluding that enhanced techniques weren't torture was contained in its memo on U.S. law, but the OLC referenced this discussion in its companion memos on international law. The Bush Administration had earlier taken the position that suspected terrorists detained by the CIA weren't subject to the Geneva Conventions.

76. Undated background paper on CIA's combined use of interrogation techniques faxed to Dan Levin at the Department of Justice, Office of Legal Counsel, on December 30, 2004, from a redacted source, http://www.aclu.org/torturefoia/released/082409/olcremand/2004olc97.pdf.

77. The collar was designed by medical personnel to reduce the risk of spinal injuries during "walling" by constraining head movement during impact with the wall.

78. Telephone interview with Michael Dunlavey, Dec. 2009.

79. See Committee, *supra* n. 38 at 38.

80. Ibid.

81. E-Mail interview with Paul Burney, March 2010.

82. See Committee, *supra* n. 38 at 40, 43–49.

83. Ibid., 45–46.

84. Percival's claimed ignorance is also contradicted by the title of one of the presentations at the training session: "Counter Measures to Defeat al Qaeda Resistance Contingency Training."

85. Jane Mayer, *The Dark Side: The Inside Story of How the War on Terror Turned into a War on American Ideals* (New York: Doubleday, 2008), 245–248.

86. Whether this happened because Banks and Percival (or other instructors at the September training session) didn't make this point or because Dr. Burney and Leso failed to grasp it remains uncertain.

87. See Committee, *supra* n. 38 at 50

88. Action Memo from William J. Haynes II, General Counsel, to Secretary of Defense, re "Counter-Resistance Techniques," dated Nov. 22, 2002 and approved by Secretary of Defense Donald Rumsfeld on Dec. 2, 2002, available at: http://www.washingtonpost.com/wp-srv/nation/documents/dodmemos.pdf

89. Paul Burney and John Leso, Memorandum for Record, Counter-Resistance Strategies, October 2, 2002, p. 1, quoted in Senate Committee on Armed Services, *Inquiry, supra* n. 38 at 52.

90. Seymour Hersh, "Torture at Abu Ghraib," *The New Yorker,* May 10, 2004, available at: www.newyorker.com/archive/2004/05/10/040510fa_fact.

91. Jonathan H. Marks, "Doctors of Interrogation," *Hastings Center Report* 35, no. 4 (2005): 17.

92. Craig Haney, Curtis Banks, & Phillip Zimbardo, "A Study of Prisoners and Guards in a Simulated Prison," *Naval Res. Reviews* (Sept. 1973): 1–17. Zimbardo's team conducted the simulation in 1971. "Guards," given no guidance on how to treat their charges, put down a rebellion by spraying inmates with fire extinguishers, stripping them naked, and putting instigators in solitary confinement. They became so abusive that Zimbardo ended the study early (and was much criticized for not stopping it even sooner). Left without limits on their behavior, participants set no boundaries of their own.

93. Uniform Code of Military Justice, 64 *Stat.* 109, art. 90 (2006).

94. See Committee, *supra* n. 38 at 63–65

Chapter Eight   Doctors as Warriors II: Ethics and Politics

1. Gregg Bloche and Jonathan H. Marks, "When Doctors Go to War," *New England Journal of Medicine* 352, no. 1 (January 6, 2005): 3–6.

2. Ibid., 4–5.

3. Eliot Friedson, *Professional Powers: A Study of the Institutionalization of Formal Knowledge* (Chicago: University of Chicago Press, 1986).

4. Shumate's formal title was "Director of Behavioral Science" for the Defense Department's Counterintelligence Field Activity. His APA task force bio boasted that he supervised a staff of twenty psychologists who provided "operational psychological support" to Pentagon agencies.

5. Report of the American Psychological Association Presidential Force on Psychological Ethics and National Security (2005), 5, www.apa.org/pubs/info/reports/pens.pdf.

6. All well and good, one might think, since "the laws of the United States" incorporate treaties that proscribe torture. And in a further feint (since the report rejected international law as a basis for defining torture), the task force said it "encourages psychologists

working in this area to review essential human rights documents," including one of these treaties, the Convention Against Torture.

7. See Report, *supra* n. 5.

8. There is some circularity here. A military order is mandatory (and disobedience is legally sanctionable) unless the order is "patently illegal"—that is, clearly contrary to military regulations or the international law of human rights and armed conflict. But U.S. military regulations (and the international law of human rights and armed conflict) require health professionals, including physicians and psychologists, to adhere to their professions' ethical obligations. So had the APA task force made adherence to "basic principles of human rights" *mandatory,* military psychologists who refused to participate in rough interrogations would have been able to argue that orders to do so were "patently illegal." But by allowing psychologists to choose "law" over "ethics," the panel made the latter *optional*—and thus not an *obligation* justifying disobedience to an order. And since the task force treated "basic principles of human rights" as "ethics," not "law," it made human rights optional—and thus an insufficient basis for disobeying an order.

   To be sure, a courageous military psychologist might have challenged the Bush administration's redefinition of torture, insisting, at a court-martial proceeding, that international law applied—as *law,* not merely *ethics.* But the psychologist's chance of prevailing would have been minimal, given the deference shown to the Justice Department's Office of Legal Counsel, which issued the torture memos.

9. The *New England Journal of Medicine* piece by Marks and me did get one detail wrong: We reported that the Guantanamo Biscuit was created by General Miller in late 2002, when, in fact, it was set up by Miller's predecessor, General Dunlavey, in June, as described in this chapter.

10. Behnke, according to a meeting participant, said that complaints to the APA about psychologists who allegedly participated in interrogation had not been accompanied by supporting evidence.

11. Pressed by military psychologists to respond quickly to charges that they'd designed and overseen torture, the APA moved with extraordinary speed. On Sunday evening Behnke and the task force's chair, Olivia Moorehead-Slaughter, sent members a draft report. Eighteen hours later, the draft was deemed final. Within a few days, the APA's Ethics Committee and Board of Directors approved the report, making only cosmetic changes. APA staff shared the report with White House and Pentagon officials in advance of its public release, which was delayed until the next Tuesday because of the July 4 weekend.

12. E-mail from Olivia Moorehead-Slaughter to listserv participants, July 29, 2005, in E-mail Messages from the Listserv of the American Psychological Association Presidential Task Force on Psychological Ethics and National Security: April 22, 2005–June 26, 2006, http://s3.amazonaws.com/propublica/assets/docs/pens_listserv.pdf

13. E-mails from Nina Thomas to listserv participants, July 29, 2005, in ibid.

14. E-mail from Gerald Koocher to listserv participants, July 30, 2005, in ibid.

15. Gerald Koocher, Open Letter to Amy Goodman [host of the syndicated talk show *Democracy Now*], excerpted in "The Empire Strikes Back: APA Tops Lash Out at Anti-Torture Opponents," *Invictus Blog,* Sept. 5, 2007, available at http://valtinsblog. blogspot.com/2007/09/empire-strikes-back-apa-tops-lash-out.html. Koocher's letter was originally posed on his own website, at: http://www.ethicsresearch.com/Open_letter_to_Amy_Goodman.pdf. As this book went to press, the letter was unavailable on Koocher's site (though the site itself was up and running)–the letter had apparently been taken down.

16. Bryce Lefever's father, Ernest, a minister in the pacifist Church of the Brethren (an Amish offshoot), wrote speeches for Hubert Humphrey during his 1960 and 1968 presidential

campaigns but shifted hard to the right thereafter. His February 1981 appointment to the post of assistant secretary of state for human rights and humanitarian affairs set off a high-profile public debate over the role of human rights in U.S. foreign policy, (Lefever insisted human rights should have no role.) And his blunt statements—for example, he called torture in Chile "a residual practice of the Iberian tradition"—led most Republicans on the Senate Foreign Relations Committee to vote against his confirmation.

17. E-mail from Gerald Koocher to listserv participants, Aug. 11, 2005, in E-mail Messages from the Listserv.

18. His examples were: "rigorous cross examination of a rape victim at a trial; interviewing convicted defendants for pre sentencing reports, interviewing sex offenders or parole candidates to determine whether their incarceration should persist; involuntary civil commitment hearings, mandated reporting of dependent person abuse, conducting independent evaluations of people claiming medical disability, profiling suspected criminals to aid in their apprehension, etc. [*sic*]."

19. American Psychiatric Association, *Psychiatric Participation in Interrogation of Detainees: Position Statement*, http://archive.psych.org/edu/other_res/lib_archives/archives/200601.pdf.

20. The association said that "psychiatrists may provide training to military or civilian investigative or law enforcement personnel on recognizing and responding to persons with mental illnesses, on the possible medical and psychological effects of particular techniques and conditions of interrogation, and on other areas within their professional expertise."

21. Michael Smith, "APA: Stay Out of Interrogations, Psychiatrists Urged," *Medpage Today*, May 22, 2006, available at www.medpagetoday.com/Psychiatry/GeneralPsychiatry/3371.

22. At some detention sites, interrogations were recorded on CDs for review by Biscuit doctors; at other sites, Biscuit doctors observed interrogations directly, through one-way mirrors.

23. By "ethical statement," he meant an ethical requirement enforceable through the association's disciplinary procedures.

24. To be sure, the psychiatry APA barred complicity in torture, but it went less far than the psychological association, which eventually defined torture by reference to international human rights principles. This, the psychiatric association didn't do.

25. *DeBlanco v. Ohio State Medical Board*, 604 N.E.2d 212 (1992).

26. Physicians for Human Rights, *Aiding Torture: Health Professionals' Ethics and Human Rights Violations Revealed in the May 2004 CIA Inspector General's Report* (2009), http://physiciansforhumanrights.org/library/documents/reports/aiding-torture.pdf

27. See Hall, *supra* chapter 1 n. 7. See also Jozien M. Bensing and William Verheul, "The Silent Healer: The Role of Communication in Placebo Effects," *Patient Education and Counseling* 80 (2010): 293–299.

28. Kenneth J. Arrow, "Uncertainty and the Welfare Economics of Medical Care," *American Economic Review* 53, no. 5 (1963): 941–973.

29. Jerrold Post, *The Psychological Assessment of Political Leaders: With Profiles of Saddam Hussein and Bill Clinton* (Ann Arbor, MI: University of Michigan Press, 2003).

30. Organisation for the Prohibition of Chemical Weapons, Convention on the Prohibition of the Development, Production, Stockpiling and Use of Chemical Weapons and on Their Destruction, April 29, 1997, available at http://www.opcw.org/chemical-weapons-convention/ . The Convention prohibits the development, production, acquisition, stockpiling, retention, transfer or use of chemical weapons by states parties–that is, by nations that have ratified the Convention.

31. Wyre Sententia, "Your Mind Is a Target: Weaponization of Psychoactive Drugs," *Humanist* 63, no 1 (2003): 43, http://web.ebscohost.com/ehost/detail?vid=1&hid=104& sid=66298062–7c8b–463f–8cd6-d98196395cdf%40sessionmgr111&bdata=JnNpdG U9ZWhvc3QtbGl2ZQ%3d%3d#db=aph&AN=871990.

32. British Medical Association, Board of Science, "The Use of Drugs as Weapons: The Concerns and Responsibilities of Healthcare Professionals" (2007), www.bma.org.uk/ images/DrugsasWeapons_tcm41–144496.pdf.

33. The position statement achieved this by defining "interrogation" as follows, so as to exclude the practice of forensic psychiatry: "As used in this statement, 'interrogation' refers to a deliberate attempt to elicit information from a detainee for the purposes of incriminating the detainee, identifying other persons who have committed or may be planning to commit acts of violence or other crimes, or otherwise obtaining information that is believed to be of value for criminal justice or national security purposes. It does not include interviews or other interactions with a detainee that have been appropriately authorized by a court or by counsel for the detainee or that are conducted by or on behalf of correctional authorities with a prisoner serving a criminal sentence."

34. Jonathan H. Marks, "Interrogational Neuroimaging in Counterterrorism: A No-Brainer or a Human Rights Hazard," *American Journal of Law and Medicine* 33, nos. 2 and 3 (2007): 483; Henry Greely and Judy Illes, "Neuroscience-Based Lie Detection: The Urgent Need for Regulation," *American Journal of Law and Medicine* 33, nos. 2 and 3 (2007): 377–431.

35. There's wide agreement among researchers in this area that neither this nor related brain scanning technologies can, so far, reliably distinguish truth from lies. More progress has been made in use of these technologies to determine whether a person being questioned recognizes, from past experience, information an interviewer gives her—a name or address, for example, or a photo of a face.

36. E.g., http://noliemri.com/customers/Government.htm.

37. Morgan, C. A., 3rd, Wang, S., Mason, J., Southwick, S. M., et al. "Hormone profiles in humans experiencing military survival training." *Biological Psychiatry* 47 (2000): 891–901.

38. For an insightful discussion of the ethics of what these authors did, see David Luban, "The Torture Lawyers of Washington," in *Legal Ethics and Human Dignity* (Cambridge: Cambridge University Press, 2007).

39. Elliot Friedson, *Profession of Medicine: A Study of the Sociology of Applied Knowledge* (Chicago: University of Chicago Press, 1988).

40. M. Gregg Bloche, "The Market for Medical Ethics," *J. Health Politics, Policy & Law* 26, no. 5 (2001):1099–1112.

Chapter Nine   Doing Justice?

1. *Washington v. Harper,* 494 U.S. 210, 222, 228 (1990).

2. Quotations from Johnson's testimony are from pre-trial Evidentiary Hearings in July, 2000. Transcript of Record, U.S. v. Russell Eugene Weston, 134 F.Supp.2d 115 (2001) (No. 98–357).

3. In a literal sense, Kramer erred: The expression, "first do no harm," is not part of the Hippocratic Oath.

4. Antonio Damasio, *Looking for Spinoza: Joy, Sorrow, and the Feeling Brain* (New York: Mariner Books, 2003).

5. Amos Tversky and Daniel Kahneman, "Judgment Under Uncertainty: Heuristics and Biases," in *Judgment under Uncertainty,* ed. Daniel Kahneman, Paul Slovic, and Amos Tversky (Cambridge, UK: Cambridge University Press, 1982).

6. *Rex v. Arnold,* 17 How. St. Tr. 695, 764 (1724).

7. *Regina v. M'Naghten,* 10 Clark and F. 200, 8 Eng. Rep. 718 (1843) (emphasis added).

8. Isaac Ray, *A Treatise on the Medical Jurisprudence of Insanity,* ed. Winfred Overholser (Cambridge, MA., Harvard University Press, 1962), 58.

9. *State v. Pike,* 49 N.H. 399, 442 (1869).

10. *Durham v. U.S.,* 214 F.2d 862 (1954).

11. American Law Institute, *Model Penal Code,* Sec. 4.01 (Proposed Official Draft) (1962) (emphasis added).

12. *U.S. v. Alexander,* 471 F.2d 923 (1973).

13. Douglas Hofstadter, *Godel, Escher, Bach: An Eternal Golden Braid,* (New York: Basic Books, 1979), 641.

14. Jamie Samuelsen, "A Rant Might Have Reversed Jim Joyce's Bad Call," *Detroit Free Press Online,* www.freep.com/article/20100910/SPORTS02/100910046/1356/SPORTS/A-rant-might-have-reversed-Jim-Joyces-bad-call.

15. Definition of the circumstances under which a person acts also involves moral judgment. The more specific we are about the circumstances–the greater the detail with which we identify social, biological, and other influences on behavior–the closer we come to absolution. Think of it this way: once we've specified every last circumstance, our causal story is complete, and *nobody* in the situation *could* have acted differently. To say that someone could have acted differently is to concede that there are causes (that is, circumstances) we are disregarding. Moral choice, in other words, inheres in our decisions about which circumstances we count and which circumstances we ignore.

16. Walter Sinnott-Armstrong ed., *The Neuroscience of Morality: Emotion, Brain Disorders, and Development* (Cambridge, MA: MIT Press, 2008); Richard Joyce, *The Evolution of Morality* (Cambridge, MA: MIT Press, 2007); Frans de Waal, *Primates and Philosophers: How Morality Evolved* (Princeton, NJ: Princeton University Press, 2006).

17. Insanity Defense Reform Act, 8 USCA § 17 (1984).

18. Transcript of record at 5, *U.S. v. Weston,* 255 F.3d 873 (D.C. Cir. 2001).

19. *U.S. v. Weston,* 255 F.3d 873, 883 (D.C. Cir. 2001).

20. Social Security Administration, Annual Statistical Report on the Social Security Disability Insurance Program, 2009 (2010), hwww.ssa.gov/policy/docs/statcomps/di_asr/.

21. Social Security Act, 42 U.S.C.A. § 423.

22. To be fair about this grossly unfair way of doing things, its proponents didn't see children as inanimate possessions; they held that fathers were better able to protect their children from life's dangers, provide for them materially, and prepare them for gainful employment as adults.

23. The "best interest of the child" standard wasn't a 1960s or 1970s invention: It had been the underlying ideal in the Anglo-American law of child custody for at least 200 years. But the sexist presumptions that prevailed into the mid-twentieth century gave it real-world content, content lost when the law dispensed with these presumptions out of concern for gender fairness.

24. Joseph Goldstein, Anna Freud, and Albert J. Solnit, *Beyond the Best Interest of the Child* (New York: Free Press, 1986).

25. Judith Areen and Milton C Regan, *Family Law: Cases and Materials* (New York: Aspen, 2006), 482–483.

26. Ibid., 506.

27. See, e.g., Jon Elster, "Solomnic Judgments: Against the Best Interest of the Child," *University of Chicago Law Review* 54, no. 1 (Winter 1987): 1–45; Robert H. Mnookin, "Child-Custody Adjudication: Judicial Functions in the Face of Indeterminacy," *Law and Contemporary Problems* 39, no. 3, Children and the Law (Summer 1975): 226–293; Andrea Charlow, "Awarding Custody: Best Interests of the Child and Other Fictions,"

Yale Law and Policy Review 5, no. 2 (Spring – Summer 1987): 267–290; Matthew B. Johnson, "Psychological Parent Theory Reconsidered: The New Jersey 'JC' Case, Part II," *American Journal of Forensic Psychology* 14, no. 2 (1999) 41, 44.

28. Joseph Goldstein "Anna Freud," *Yale Law Journal* 92, no. 2 (1982), 219, 221 – 222.

29. Ibid., 221.

30. Ibid., 220.

31. Ibid., 221.

32. See, e.g., Michael Lamb, "The Emergent American Father" in *The Father's Role: Cross-Cultural Perspectives,* ed. Michael E. Lamb (Hillsdale, NJ: Lawrence Earlbaum Associates, Inc., 1987): 3–23; Marshall L. Hamilton, *Father's Influence on Children* (Chicago: Nelson Hall Publishers, 1977).

33. Michael Lamb, "How Do Fathers Influence Children's Development? Let Me Count the Ways," in *The Role of the Father in Child Development,* ed. Michael Lamb (Hoboken, NJ: Wiley, 2010), 1–26.

34. Judith A. Seltzer et al., "Family Ties After Divorce: The Relationship Between Visiting and Paying Child Support," *Journal of Marriage and the Family* 51 (1989): 1013 – 1014.

35. For the better part of the twentieth century, federal and state courts required that expert testimony be based on techniques "generally accepted" in the relevant scientific community. In 1993, the U.S. Supreme Court tightened federal standards for admission of experts' conclusions, mandating that they qualify as scientific knowledge, derived from "scientific methodology." *Daubert v. Merrell Dow Pharmaceuticals,* 509 U.S. 579 (1993). More than half of the states have adopted variations on this approach.

36. Robert E. Emery, Randy K Otto, William T. O'Donohue, "A Critical Assessment of Child Custody Evaluations: Limited Science and a Flawed System," *Psychological Science in the Public Interest* 6 no. 1 (2005) 1–29; Daniel W. Shuman, "The Role of Mental Health Experts in Custody Decisions: Science, Psychological Tests, and Clinical Judgment," *Family Law Quarterly* 36 (2002) 135–162; Daniel A. Krauss and Bruce D. Sales, "Legal Standards, Expertise, and Experts in the Resolution of Contested Child Custody Cases," *Psychology, Public Policy, and Law* 6 no. 4 (2000) 843–879.

37. Timothy M. Tippins and Jeffrey P. Wittmann, "Empirical and Ethical Problems with Custody Recommendations: A Call for Clinical Humility and Judicial Vigilance," *Family Court Review* 43 no. 2 (2005): 193.

38. Separating spouses can generally avoid a custody evaluation by agreeing to a parenting schedule on their own.

39. There've been no systematic studies of the influence of psychiatrists' and psychologists' custody evaluations on litigation outcomes. The difficulty of acquiring and reviewing a meaningful sample of court records probably precludes such an inquiry: There is no centralized reporting system for such cases, and litigation records are often "sealed" (i.e., made secret) by court order after the proceedings to protect the privacy of the parties. Nor have there been empirical studies of how custody evaluations influence settlements. The confidentiality of these evaluations, absent trial proceedings that reveal their content, makes such studies impossible. But the folk wisdom among divorce lawyers and custody evaluators with whom I've spoken is that an evaluation entered into evidence at trial is very difficult to "beat" (so long as the evaluator was agreed to by both parties) and that this drives parties to agree to parenting schedules pretty close to what evaluators recommend.

40. There is no scientific evidence that training in psychiatry or clinical psychology enhances people's ability to detect deception or to parse through contradictory claims to find the truth.

41. These several reports didn't come my way in random fashion; they were offered by custody litigants who objected to them. I thus make no claim that they're representative in

any statistical sense. Rigorous empirical study of the extent to which custody evaluators base their recommendations on cultural biases, contested moral premises, and their own answers to disputed questions of fact would require access to a statistically meaningful sample of evaluation reports, obtained in random fashion. Such access is unlikely.

42. "Fred" and "Ally" are pseudonyms, as are the names I've employed for their children and for mental health professionals who participated in their case; I've also changed some geographic details. "Ally," who shared custody evaluations from her case with me for this book, gave me permission to use her real name but asked me to otherwise preserve her family's anonymity. To ensure their anonymity, I've employed a pseudonym for "Ally" as well; "Ally" has given me permission to do so.

43. Weekday time was a battleground because weekends with Dad could be done as visits—he could go to Washington to see the children or they could go to New Jersey—while weekday residence with both parents would require them to live nearby.

44. *Stenberg v. Carhart,* 11 F. Supp. 2d 1099 (Neb. 1998).

45. *Stenberg v. Carhart,* 530 U.S. 914 (2000).

46. Partial Birth Abortion Ban Act, 18 U.S.C. § 1531(2003).

47. More precisely, the statute included a congressional "finding" that "moral, medical, and ethical consensus exists that . . . partial birth abortion . . . is a gruesome and inhumane procedure that is never medically necessary." This "finding" was, of course, untrue—there was no such consensus. Physicians had lined up on both sides of the medical necessity question, and the medical specialty organization representing gynecologists had taken the position that the procedure was sometimes necessary. But the courts have long given great deference to legislative fact-finding.

48. The Supreme Court also held that Congress had defined the term "partial birth abortion" with sufficient specificity, something that (according to the justices) the Nebraska legislature didn't do.

49. C. Lanni et al., "Cognition Enhancers Between Treating and Doping the Mind," *Pharmacological Research* 57 no. 3 (2008): 196–213.

50. Henry Greely, Barbara Sahakian, et al., "Toward Responsible Use of Cognitive-Enhancing Drugs by the Healthy," *Nature* 456 (2008): 702–705.

51. The American Psychiatric Association's *DSM-IV,* almost universally followed, at least in form, by doctors who diagnosis ADHD on the basis of "inattention," requires a finding that "six (or more) of the following symptoms of inattention have persisted for at least 6 months to a degree that is maladaptive and inconsistent with developmental level":

- often fails to give close attention to details or makes careless mistakes in schoolwork, work, or other activities
- often has difficulty sustaining attention in tasks or play activities
- often does not seem to listen when spoken to directly
- often does not follow through on instructions and fails to finish schoolwork, chores, or duties in the workplace (not due to oppositional behavior or failure to understand instructions)
- often has difficulty organizing tasks and activities
- often avoids, dislikes, or is reluctant to engage in tasks that require sustained mental effort (such as schoolwork or homework)
- often loses things necessary for tasks or activities (e.g., toys, school assignments, pencils, books, or tools)
- is often easily distracted by extraneous stimuli
- is often forgetful in daily activities.

See *Diagnostic and Statistical Manual, supra* chapter 5 n. 1 at 92.

52. They must also be "inconsistent with developmental level," a prerequisite that's less restrictive than meets the eye. True, distractibility that's age-appropriate for toddlers isn't for teens, but people vary so widely in their concentration and attention to detail that there aren't well-defined "developmental levels" for these traits, allowing doctors wide discretion on this front.

53. Work by Nobel laureate Eric Kandel and others has shown that long-term memory (i.e., memory lasting longer than a few hours) forms when chemical signals enter nerve cell nuclei, triggering the expression of genes that produce proteins, which, in turn, create new intercellular connections and other structures. This work opens the way for pharmaceutical interventions to block these chemical pathways.

54. "Mecca Thief Has His Hand Cut Off," BBC News, October 27, 2002, http://news.bbc. co.uk/2/hi/middle_east/2366419.stm; "Iran Court Orders 'Eye for an Eye' Blinding of Road Rage Man" Al Bawaba News, August 21, 2000, www1.albawaba.com/en/news/ iran-court-orders-eye-eye-blinding-road-rage-man.

55. Atul Gawande, "When Law and Ethics Collide—Why Physicians Participate in Executions," *New England Journal of Medicine* 354, no.12 (2006): 1221, 1226.

56. Mary Ann Farkas and Gale Miller, "Sex Offender Treatment: Reconciling Criminal Justice Priorities and Therapeutic Goals," *Federal Sentencing Reporter* 21 no. 2 (December 2008): 78–82.

57. *State of Louisiana v. Perry,* 610 So. 2d 746 (1992).

58. Perry's case followed a circuitous legal path: His appeal made it all the way to the U.S. Supreme Court, which agreed to hear the case, then declined to decide it, instead remanding it to the trial court for reconsideration.

59. *Singleton v. State,* 313 S.C. 75, 437 S.E. 2d 53 (1993).

60. *Singleton v. Norris,* 319 F.3d 1018 (2003).

61. *Washington v. Glucksberg,* 521 U.S. 702 (1997) (*en banc*).

62. *Singleton v. Norris,* 319 F.3d 1018 (8th Cir. 2003), *cert denied,* 540 U.S. 832 (2003).

63. *Sell v. U.S.,* 539 U.S. 166 (2003).

64. Prosecutors had to show a court that "important governmental interests are at stake"—the likelihood of long-term psychiatric confinement meant that the government's interest in prosecuting crimes counted for less. Prosecutors also had to prove that the drugs were both likely to restore competence and unlikely to have disabling side effects. And they had to show that "alternative, less intrusive treatments" are unlikely to achieve this result.

65. *Baze v. Rees,* 553 U.S. 35 (2008).

66. Ibid., at 67 (Alito, J., concurring).

67. Deborah W. Denno, "The Lethal Injection Quandary: How Medicine Has Dismantled the Death Penalty," *Fordham Law Review* 76 no. 1 (2007): 49.

68. The court in *Washington v. Glucksberg* invoked the state's interest in preserving life and the historical unlawfulness of suicide, among other factors. And looming over the assisted suicide debate was the loaded question of abortion—many who backed the constitutionality of laws restricting abortion saw support for laws against assisted suicide as a sign of pro-life bona fides.

69. Formally, the lawyer (known as a guardian *ad litem*) represented the children in the litigation. Her practical role was to conduct a separate inquiry (interviewing the same therapists and family members questioned by the custody evaluators) and to make her own custody recommendation to the court.

70. Paul Appelbaum, "The Parable of the Forensic Psychiatrist: Ethics and the Problem of Doing Harm," *International Journal of Law and Psychiatry* 13 no. 4 (1990): 249, 252.

Chapter Ten   Conclusion

1. Telephone interview with Vikram Kapil, Oct. 2010.
2. Over the previous several years, Virginia ranked second only to Texas in annual executions.
3. Telephone interview with Daniel Zwerdling, Oct. 2010.
4. National Public Radio, *All Things Considered*, "The Role of Physicians in Executions," April 3, 1994. Transcript available at http://nl.newsbank.com/nl-search/we/Archives?p_action=doc&p_docid=0F574EA799B24146&p_docnum=1&s_dlid=DL0111011117424801762&s_ecproduct=SUB-FREE&s_ecprodtype=INSTANT&s_trackval=&s_siteloc=&s_referrer=&s_subterm=Subscription%20until%3A%2012%2F14%2F2015%2011%3A59%20PM&s_docsbal=%20&s_subexpires=12%2F14%2F2015%2011%3A59%20PM&s_docstart=&s_docsleft=&s_docsread=&s_username=freeuser&s_accountid=AC0109083112065524669&s_upgradeable=no
5. Ibid.
6. Ibid.
7. David Lerman, "Debating Ethics on Death Row: Executions Trouble Top Prison Doctor," *Daily Press*, April 6, 1994, http://articles.dailypress.com/1994–04–06/news/9404060074_1_future-executions-southside-strangler-death-row
8. During the weeks after the NPR taping, as his views on pronouncing death (and dealing with the governor's reaction) evolved, Dr. Kapil kept in touch with me periodically by phone. The account herein is based on what Kapil told me, his son Vikram's recollections, and contemporary press reports.
9. M. Gregg Bloche and Leslie A. Meltzer, eds., *Antidote: Strategies for Containing America's Runaway Health Care Costs* (The Brookings Institution Press, forthcoming).
10. Even the lawyers challenging the constitutionality of lethal injection conceded its near painlessness when properly administered. Their arguments focused on the possibility of suffering if things go wrong (e.g., poor IV placement or a barbiturate dose that's not enough to make the condemned unconscious before he's given the drugs that stop breathing and heart function).
11. James Glanz and Alan Schwarz, "From 'Avatar' Playbook, Athletes Use 3-D Imaging," *New York Times*, October 2, 2010, http://www.nytimes.com/2010/10/03/sports/03reality.html?_r=1&scp=11&sq=james+glanz&st=nyt
12. Ibid.
13. Dan Larriviere, "Responding to Requests from Adult Patients for Neuroenhancements: Guidance of the Ethics, Law, and Humanities Committee," *Neurology* 73, no. 17 (2009): 1406–1412.
14. Martha J. Farah et al., "Neurocognitive Enhancement: What Can We Do and What Should We Do?" *Nature Reviews: Neuroscience* 5 (2004): 421–425.
15. Robert Frank, "Social Norms as Positional Arms Control Agreements," in *Economics, Values, and Organization,* ed. Avner Ben-Ner and Louis Putterman (Cambridge, UK: Cambridge University Press, 1998), 275–295.

index